Filipe Natalio

Marine Biomaterials

Filipe Natalio

Marine Biomaterials

Bioinspired fabrication of biosilica-based bone substitution materials

Südwestdeutscher Verlag für Hochschulschriften

Imprint
Any brand names and product names mentioned in this book are subject to trademark, brand or patent protection and are trademarks or registered trademarks of their respective holders. The use of brand names, product names, common names, trade names, product descriptions etc. even without a particular marking in this work is in no way to be construed to mean that such names may be regarded as unrestricted in respect of trademark and brand protection legislation and could thus be used by anyone.

Publisher:
Südwestdeutscher Verlag für Hochschulschriften
is a trademark of
Dodo Books Indian Ocean Ltd., member of the OmniScriptum S.R.L Publishing group
str. A.Russo 15, of. 61, Chisinau-2068, Republic of Moldova Europe
Printed at: see last page
ISBN: 978-3-8381-1934-2

Zugl. / Approved by: Mainz, JGU, Diss., 2010

Copyright © Filipe Natalio
Copyright © 2010 Dodo Books Indian Ocean Ltd., member of the OmniScriptum S.R.L Publishing group

Bioinspired fabrication of biosilica-based bone substitution materials

Dissertation
zur Erlangung des Grades
Doktor der Naturwissenschaften
im Promotionsfach Chemie

Am Fachbereich Chemie, Pharmazie und Geowissenschaften
der Johannes Gutenberg-Universität
in Mainz

Filipe André da Silva Raminhos Natálio
geb. in Caldas da Rainha (Portugal)

Mainz, 13th July 2010

To my parents
Raquel e Joãozinho

Index

1. Summary/Zusammenfassung..8

2. Introduction
2.1. Biomineralization..12
2.2. Sponges as Eumetazoa: A long pathway...............................14
2.3. Biomineralization in sponges......................................15
    2.3.1. Geological background..15
    2.3.2. Biosilification in spicules....................................15
        2.3.2.1. Structural features......................................15
        2.3.2.2. Biochemical approach.....................................16
        2.3.2.3. Silicatein – Silica polymerizing protein.................16
        2.3.2.4. Spiculogenesis...17
2.4. Silicatein wide applications......................................21
    2.4.1. Bionanotechnological applications of silicatein................21
    2.4.2. Biomedical approach..23
2.5. Calcium Phosphate biominerals.....................................25
    2.5.1. Bone..25
        2.5.1.1. Bone has functional biomineral in animal evolution......25
        2.5.1.2. Bone hierarchial composition............................26
        2.5.1.2. Bone biomineralization..................................27
2.6. Tissue engineering..30
    2.6.1. Overview..30
    2.6.2. Biological/medical approach....................................31
        2.6.2.1. Bone grafts...31
    2.6.3. Synthetic and biomimetic materials.............................32
        2.6.3.1. Silica containing implant: Bioglass®....................34

3. Experimental Procedure

3.1. Component A: Microencapsulation of silicatein and respective precursor into poly(D,L-lactide) biodegradable microspheres..........................37

    3.1.1. Production of polymeric spheres containing both silicatein and silica..37

    3.1.2. Physical characterization of PLA microspheres...............................37

        3.1.2.1. Microscopic analysis of the PLA-silicatein microspheres...37

        3.1.2.2. Dynamic Light Scattering (DLS)..............................38

    3.1.3. Immunodetection of encapsulated silicatein................................38

        3.1.3.1. Immunoblotting...38

        3.1.3.2. Immunochemistry..39

    3.1.4. Elemental detection of encapsulated silica...................................39

    3.1.5. Release of silicatein from polymeric microsphere.........................39

    3.1.6. Enzyme linked Immunosorbent assay (ELISA)...........................40

    3.1.7. Determination of enzymatic activity..41

3.2. Component B: Production of plastic-like filler matrix containing silicic acid (PMSA)..41

    3.2.1. Plastic-like filler matrix containing silicic acid (PMSA)................41

    3.2.2. Microscopic analysis of the plastic-like filler matrix (PMSA)............42

    3.2.3. X-ray diffraction (XRD) of the plastic-like filler matrix (PMSA)........42

3.3. Bifunctional 2-component implant..42

    3.3.1. Physical properties of bifunctional 2-component implant................42

        3.3.1.1. Hardness measurements..42

        3.3.1.2. Bifunctional 2-component implant behavior in simulated body fluid (SBF)..42

        3.3.1.3. Release/adhesion of silicatein to bifunctional 2-component implant: Immunochemistry.....................43

       3.3.1.4. Adhesion of silicatein to bifunctional 2-component
       implant: Fourier Transform Infrared spectroscopy with
       attenuated total reflection (FT-IR ATR) for
       protein-surface interaction......43

       3.3.1.5. Imaging properties on bifunctional
       2-component implant......43

  3.3.2. Cell proliferation assay on bifunctional
      2-component implant......43

3.4. Animal experiments......44

  3.4.1. Surgery and implantation......44

  3.4.2. Computed tomography (CT) and
      micro-computed tomography (μ-CT) analysis......45

4. Results......47

4.1. Component A: Microencapsulation of silicatein and silica precursor (sodium metasilicate) into poly(D,L-lactide) biodegradable microspheres......47

  4.1.1. Production of polymeric spheres containing both
      silicatein and silica......47

  4.1.2. Physical characterization of PLA microspheres......48

  4.1.3. Immunodetection of encapsulated silicatein......49

      4.1.3.1. Dot-blot......49

      4.1.3.2. Thin cuts......51

  4.1.4. Detection of encapsulated silica source......53

  4.1.5. Release of silicatein from polymeric microspheres......54

  4.1.6. Determination of enzymatic activity......56

4.2. Component B: Production of plastic-like filler matrix containing silicic acid (PMSA)......57

  4.2.1. Preparation of a plastic-like filler matrix
      containing silicic acid (PMSA)......57

4.3. Bifunctional 2-component implant...59
    4.3.1. Physical properties of bifunctional 2-component
    implant: Hardness measurements...59
    4.3.2. Bifunctional 2-component implant in
    simulated body fluid (SBF)...61
    4.3.3. Release and adhesion of silicatein
    onto the bifunctional 2-component implant......................................61
    4.3.4. Imaging properties of bifunctional 2-component implant...............65
    4.3.5. Cytoxicity assay...65
4.4. Animal experiments..67
    4.4.1. Surgery and implantation...67
    4.4.2. Computed tomography (CT) and
    micro-computed tomography (μ-CT) analysis of
    implant contrast within the bone..68
    4.4.3. Analysis of bone regenerative capacity
    after 9 weeks of implantation..71
        4.4.3.1. External Morphology...71
        4.4.3.2. Computed tomography (CT).......................................73

5. Discussion..75
**5.1. Microencapsulation of silicatein and respective precursor
(sodium metasilicate) into poly(D,L-lactide)
biodegradable microspheres**...76
5.2. Release of silicatein from polymeric microspheres (PLASSM)..................80
**5.3. Component B: Production of plastic-like filler
matrix containing silicic acid (PMSA)**..82
5.4. Bifunctional 2-component implant..85
    5.4.1. Cytoxicity studies..88
5.5. Bifunctional 2-component implant: *ex vivo* and *in vivo* studies................89
    5.5.1. *Ex vivo* studies..89
    5.5.2. *In vivo* preliminary studies..90

6. Conclusion..93

7. Bibliography...94

8. List of abbreviations..110

1. Summary

Until today, autogenic bone grafts from various donor regions represent the gold standard in the field of bone reconstruction, providing both osteoinductive and osteoconductive characteristics. However, due to low availability and a disequilibrium between supply and demand, the risk of disease transfer and morbidity, usually associated with autogeneic bone grafts, the development of biomimic materials with structural and chemical properties similar to those of natural bone have been extensively studied. So far, only a few synthetic materials, so far, have met these criteria, displaying properties that allow an optimal bone reconstitution. Biosilica is formed enzymatically under physiological-relevant conditions (temperature and pH) via silicatein (silica protein), an enzyme that was isolated from siliceous sponges, cloned, and prepared in a recombinant way, retaining its catalytic activity. It is biocompatible, has some unique mechanical characteristics, and comprises significant osteoinductive activity.

To explore the application of biosilica in the fields of regenerative medicine, silicatein was encapsulated, together with its substrate sodium metasilicate, into poly(D,L-lactide)/polyvinylpyrrolidone(PVP)-based microspheres, using w/o/w methodology with solvent casting and termed Poly(D,L-lactide)-silicatein-silica-containing-microspheres [PLASSM]. Both silicatein encapsulation efficiency (40%) and catalytic activity retention upon polymer encapsulation were enhanced by addition of an essential pre-emulsifying step using PVP. Furthermore, the metabolic stability, cytoxicity as well as the kinetics of silicatein release from the PLASSM were studied under biomimetic conditions, using simulated body fluid. As a solid support for PLASSM, a polyvinylpyrrolidone/starch/Na_2HPO_4-based matrix (termed plastic-like filler matrix containing silicic acid [PMSA]) was developed and its chemical and physical properties determined. Moreover, due to the non-toxicity and bioactivity of the PMSA, it is suggested that PMSA acts as osteoconductive material.

Both components, PLASSM and PMSA, when added together, form a bifunctional 2-component implant material, that is (i) non-toxic (biocompatible), (ii) moldable, (iii) self-hardening at a controlled and clinically suitable rate to allows a tight insertion into any bone defect (iv) biodegradable, (v) forms a porous material upon exposure to body biomimetic conditions, and (vi) displays both osteoinductive (silicatein) and osteoconductive (PMSA) properties.

Preliminary *in vivo* experiments were carried out with rabbit femurs, by creating artificial bone defects that were subsequently treated with the bifunctional 2-component implant material. After 9 weeks of implantation, both computed tomography (CT) and morphological analyses showed complete resorption of the implanted material, concurrent with complete bone regeneration. The given data can be considered as a significant contribution to the successful introduction of biosilica-based implants into the field of bone substitution surgery.

1. Zusammenfassung

Autogenetische Knochentransplantate von verschiedenen Spenderregionen stellen bis heute den höchsten Stand auf dem Gebiet der Knochenrekonstruktion dar, indem sie sowohl osteoinduktive als auch osteokonduktive Charakteristika aufweisen. Deren geringe Verfügbarkeit, die Unausgewogenheit zwischen Angebot und Nachfrage, und die normalerweise von autogenetischen Knochentransplantaten ausgehende Ansteckungs- und Erkrankungsgefahr haben jedoch zur Entwicklung von biomimetischen Materialien geführt, die aufgrund ihrer strukturellen und chemischen Eigenschaften stark denen natürlicher Knochen ähneln. Soweit konnten allerdings nur einige wenige synthetische Materialien diese Kriterien erfüllen, da deren Eigenschaften eine optimale Knochenrekonstruktion erlauben. Biosilica wird unter physiologisch-relevanten Bedingungen (Temperatur und pH-Wert) mit Hilfe von Silicatein (Silica Protein) enzymatisch gebildet. Bei Letzterem handelt es sich um ein aus Silikat-Schwämmen isoliertes, kloniertes und rekombinant aufbereitetes Enzym, das katalytische Aktivität aufweist. Biosilica ist biologisch verträglich, hat einzigartige mechanische Eigenschaften und besitzt eine bedeutende osteoinduktive Aktivität.

Um die Anwendung von Biosilica auf dem Gebiet der regenerativen Medizin zu erforschen, wurde Silicatein zusammen mit seinem Substrat Sodium-Metasilikat in Mikrosphären eingekapselt, die auf Poly(D,L-Lactid)/Polyvinylpyrrolidon (PVP) basieren. Dies erfolgte unter Einsatz der w/o/w Methode durch Gießen von Lösungsmittel und führte zur Bezeichnung Poly(D,L-Lactid)-Silikatein-Silica-enthaltende Mikrosphären [PLASSM]. Durch einen weiteren essentiellen Schritt vor der Emulgierung mittels PVP wurde sowohl die Effizienz der Silicatein-Einkapselung (40%) als auch die Aufrechterhaltung seiner katalytischen Aktivität mittels Polymereinkapselung gesteigert. Durch den Einsatz von simulierter Körperflüssigkeit wurde darüber hinaus die metabolische Stabilität, die Zytotoxizität als auch die Kinetik der Silicatein-Freisetzung aus den PLASSM unter biomimetischen Bedingungen untersucht. Als Stützpunkt für die PLASSM wurde eine auf Polyvinylpyrrolidon/Stärke/Na_2HPO-basierende Matrix entwickelt, deren chemische sowie auch physikalische Eigenschaften daraufhin bestimmt wurden. Diese Plastik-ähnliche Füllmatrix enthält Kieselsäure und wird somit kurz PMSA genannt. PMSA scheint sogar durch seine fehlende Toxizität und seine biologische Trägheit als osteokonduktives Material zu agieren.

Wenn beide Komponenten, PLASSM und PMSA, gemeinsam hinzugefügt werden, bilden sie ein bifunktionelles, aus Zwei-Komponenten bestehendes Material für Implantate, das (i) nichttoxisch (biokompatibel), (ii) formbar und (iii) zu einem kontrollierbarem sowie klinisch-angemessenem Grad selbst-härtend ist, um es auf stabile Weise bei Knochendefekten jeder Art einzusetzen. Darüber hinaus ist es (iv) biologisch abbaubar, (v) wandelt sich nach Exposition zu Bedingungen, wie sie im Körper vorkommen, in ein poröses Material um und (vi) weist sowohl osteoinduktive (Silicatein) als auch osteokonduktive (PMSA) Eigenschaften auf.

Vorläufige *in vivo* Experimente wurden an Hasen-Femora ausgeführt, indem künstliche Knochenschäden hervorgerufen wurden, die anschließend mit dem neuen Implantat-Material behandelt wurden. Neun Wochen nach der Implantation zeigten sowohl Computertomographie (CT) als auch morphologische Analysen eine vollständige Resorption des eingepflanzten Materials sowie gleichzeitig eine komplette Regeneration des Knochens. Die in dieser Arbeit erhaltenen Daten können als ein bedeutender Beitrag zur erfolgreichen Einführung von Biosilica-enthaltenden Implantaten in das Gebiet der Knochenersatz-Chirurgie betrachtet werden.

2. Introduction

2.1. Biomineralization

During animal evolution biomolecules (e.g., secondary metabolites) and biomaterials (e.g., biominerals) were selected for higher biological efficiency and superior physical properties.[1] Pioneers in exploiting secondary metabolites for biomedical applications outlined strategies to discover and apply bioactive compounds in biomedical field, resulting in the development of 9-ß-D arabinofuranosyladenosine (ara-A) as a first active pharmaceutical ingredient.[2] Exploitation of biominerals was pioneered by Lowenstam and Weiner [3], who introduced the first extensive and comprehensive description of inorganic mineral formation within organisms highlithing the fundamental importance of organic macromolecules during biomineralization. These authors classified biominerals into two categories: (i) biologically induced mineralization and (ii) biologically controlled mineralization. (Figure 1)

In a typical inorganic mineral formation (in chemical terms), the conversion of monomers (e.g., metals or their salts) into solid state material usually occurs through endothermic reactions. The products are characterized by a defined chemical composition/physical structure and can be amorphous or crystalline. For example, quartz [SiO_2] is formed in aqueous solution under high temperatures and often high pressures (e.g. geological environments) and the crystal growth proceeds by progressive layered deposition of dissolved orthosilicic acid [H_4SiO_4] on its surface. (Figure 1 A)

In contrast to its inorganic counter part, biomineral formation combines the use inorganic and organic matrices, i.e., biologically induced mineralization. In this case during seeding phase, particles/aggregates or organisms surface containing organic biomolecules (polymers and proteins) allow nucleation and crystal growth in a non-controlled fashion.[4] For example, calcitic remains of single-celled algae, coccolithophorids and/or coccolithospheres, have been recently shown to have mineralization activity in the deep sea formation of ferromanganese crusts.[5] (Figure 1B)

On the other hand, biologically controlled mineralization is a process that occurs inside and/or outside organisms that use biomolecules to control precise initiation, growth and morphology of minerals. Biominerals can be also classified as composite materials (e.g. biocomposites) formed from the inorganic mineral and the organic component (e.g. biomolecules) with unique and remarkable properties. Interesting to note that the organic component plays a dual role in biologically controlled mineralization function both as seeds and also as scaffolds during subsequent growing phases.[4]

Introduction

A special form of biologically controlled mineralization has been described for the biosilicification process in diatoms and siliceous sponges.[6,7] (Figure 1 C and D) In marine sponges (Demospongiae and Hexactinellida) an enzyme named silicatein (silica protein) catalyzes the formation of biosilica [7,8,9] serving also as an organic scaffold, [10,11] where in diatoms poly-silicate mineral formation is passive, i.e., silica deposition is mediated by interaction of positively charged polymers (sillafins) and inorganic negatively charged orthosilicic acid [H_4SiO_4].[12] Within the view of using Nature as an inspirational source and the discovery of organic molecules that implicated in the formation of biominerals, a paradigm shift in biomaterials science and technology was created, leading to concept of fabricating synthetic biominerals with exquisite and distinguished (bio)chemical and (bio)physical properties.[13]

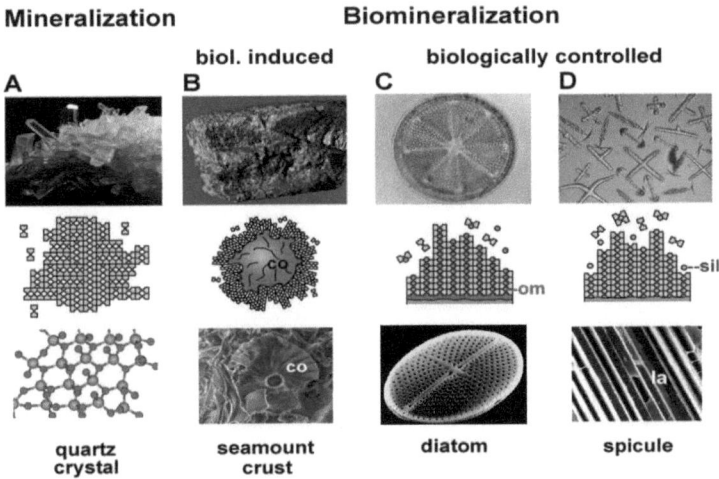

Figure 1. Mineralization.*vs*.biomineralization. (**A**) Mineralization process: quartz crystal formation. (**B**) Biologically Induced Mineralization: ferromanganese crust formation in the deep sea. Coccospheres (co) of biogenic origin serve as organic template for mineral deposition. (**C**) Biologically Controlled Mineralization: example frustule formation in the diatom *Cyclotella antigua*. Bio-seeds and organic matrices (organic guiding macromolecule [om]) control initiation and growth of the biomineral. (**D**) Of Biologically Controlled Mineralization: spicule formation in the hexactinellid *Hyalonema mirabile*.

2.2. Sponges as Eumetazoa: A long pathway

Sponges are aquatic, sessile and multicellular organisms with a body plan (Bauplan) apparently simple lacking morphological similarities to any other organisms. In early studies, sponges had been classified as "Zoophyta" [14] or "Thierpflanzen".[15] However, it was Grant who first grouped sponges into a common taxon, termed "phylum Porifera".[16] The discovery of glass sponges (class Hexactinellida), [17] broadened the definition of sponges "as sessile, marine animals with a soft and spongy (amorphously shaped) body" to include "most strongly individualized, radially symmetrical" entities.[18]

Later on, with the discovery of significant cellular morphological similarities between a highly differentiated poriferan cell type (choanocytes) and unicellular flagellate eukaryotes (choanoflagellates) a close relationship between the phyla Porifera and Choanozoa was established.[19,20] In more recent years, several molecules have been isolated, cloned and phylogenetically analyzed showing its high homology with higher metazoans becoming obvious that the phylum Porifera forms the basis of the metazoan kingdom.[21] Recently, it was finally clarified that the three classes of sponges, Hexactinellida (glass sponges), Demospongiae (silicate/spongin sponges), and Calcarea (calcareous sponges) are monophyletic and closely related to the common ancestor of all metazoans, the Urmetazoa.[22] (Figure 2)

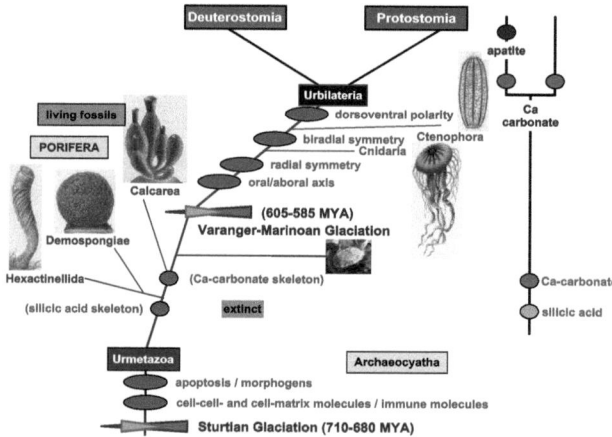

Figure 2. Phlyogenetic position of the Porifera between the Urmetazoa and the Urbilateria. The major evolutionary novelties which must be attributed to the Urmetazoa are those molecules which mediate apoptosis and control morphogenesis, the immune molecules, and primarily the cell adhesion molecules.

2.3. Biomineralization in sponges

2.3.1. Geological background

Neoproterozoic oceans were saturated in silicic acid and carbonates that were continuously introduced by weathering cycles. Consequently, it is easily conceivable why animals integrated silica and carbonate as their fundamental element for building-up their inorganic skeleton.[23] However, there is no clear explanation so far for organism elemental speciation.

In order to understand sponge biomineralization process it was necessary to track back its origins. Sponge fossil records showed that these animals first appeared during Neoproterozoic (1,000 to 542 Ma).[24, 25] During this period also other multicellular animals existed, which became extinct, [26] especially during the Varanger-Marinoan ice ages (605 to 585 Ma). Sponges were able to successful overcome big Earth events, such as several ice ages mainly due to major reasons: (i) symbiosis with microorganisms and (ii) presence of hard skeletons.[25] The maintenance of symbiotic relationships with microorganisms (e.g. bacteria) within its sophisticated aquiferous canal system allowed sponges to survive adverse environmental conditions because these autotrophic symbionts represented rich organic carbon sources. Additionally, the development of skeletal elements facilitated size increment, a common metazoan phyletic trend also known as Cope's Rule.[27]

2.3.2. Biosilification in spicules

2.3.2.1. Structural features

Skeletal elements (spicules) of siliceous sponges (e.g. Hexactinellida and Demospongiae) are composed of amorphous opal ($SiO_2 \cdot nH_2O$) with different shapes and sizes reaching up to 2.5m.[28] The immense diversity on sponge spicules shapes found within these three classes has been extensively described since the beginning of illustrative works developed by Gesner in 1558 [29] and its microscopic analysis has been considered as reliable and common classification method for sponge biologists. [for review see 30 and references herein]. Although physical and chemical analysis of spicules was performed, it was concluded that the inorganic matrix (amorphous opal) is almost indistinguishable among the studied spicules.[31] At the same time, it was demonstrated that spicules of the demosponge *T. aurantium*, after etching of spicular cross-sections, are composed of silica nanoparticles, with a mean diameter of 75 nm, tightly packed forming a compact layers separated by a organic layer.[32] Later on, Woesz et al. provided Raman spectroscopy evidence for the existence of proteins between siliceous layers (e.g. organic interlayers in *M. chun* spicule).[33] Using High

Resolution Scanning Electron Microscopy (HRSEM), Atomic Force Microscopy (AFM) and a biochemical approach it has been suggested that proteins are localized, not only between the interlamellar structure but also within the siliceous layers.[34] It was concluded that the unique combination of mechanical properties, such as strength, stiffness and toughness observed in hexactinellid spicules is based on the organic components localized within.[13]

2.3.2.2. Biochemical approach

It took until 1999 when Cha et al. discovered that one of the constituents of the filament, located within the axial canal of spicules from *Tethya aurantium*, is an enzyme, subsequently termed silicatein (silica protein), which is involved in biosilica formation.[8] Despite the fact that the same author proposed an enzymatic reaction mechanism of silicatein it took until very recently confirm experimentally the detailed properties of the reaction kinetics.[35]

Soon after having identified this ANABOLIC ENZYME, the corresponding CATABOLIC ENZYME (silicase) was also discovered. The identification of a biosilica degrading enzyme supported the view that the siliceous components in spicules are dynamic processes of building-dissolution-building cycles, in a similar way to other biominerals such as bones and teeth.[36]

2.3.2.3. Silicatein – Silica polymerizing protein

The corresponding deduced silicatein polypeptide comprises about 325 amino acids [aa] with a molecular weight of ca. 35 kDa. During maturation, the primary translation product (proenzyme) is processed by cleaving off a signal peptide (aa_1 to aa_{17}; *Suberites domuncula* [demosponge] silicatein-α) and the adjacent propeptide (aa_{18} to aa_{112}), resulting in the mature enzyme that has a size of 24-25 kDa. It could also be demonstrated that silicatein exists not only in the axial canal but also in the extraspicular and extra-cellular space.[9]

Similar to cathepsins, the catalytic center of silicatein contains histidine (His), serine (Ser) and asparagine (Asn). However, the cysteine (Cys) of the cathepsins' catalytic triad is exchanged by serine (Ser) in silicatein. In addition to about 10 putative protein kinase phosphorylation sites, silicateins display a cluster of serine residues (3x Ser) that is found close to the central amino acid residues (His, Ser and Asn) of the catalytic triad which is absent in cathepsins. Subsequent phylogenetic analyses revealed that silicateins form a separate branch from cathepsins.[7] The difficult accessibility of hexactinellids, which live primarily in depths of more than 300 m, generally results in very poor sampling. Only recently the first hexactinellid silicatein (*Crateromorpha meyeri*) could be identified and characterized.[37] This molecule shares high similarity to the demosponge sequences (expect-value

Introduction

of $8e^{-58}$) and contains the same catalytic triad amino acids. However, striking in the *C. meyeri* sequence is a second Ser-rich cluster, which is located between the second and the third amino acids of the catalytic triad. Strong binding of the protein to the spicule silica surface has been attributed to this cluster.[10]

The post-translational modifications of silicatein have been found to be essential for the enzyme activity with respect to (*i*) association with other structural and functional molecules within the tissue [38] and (*ii*) self-association/self-assembly. Fractal structures derived from silicatein self-assembled oligomers have been described for both demosponges *T. aurantium*, [39] *S. domuncula* [40] and hexactinellids (*M. chuni*).[11] Silicatein was isolated from spicules using glycerol-based buffer and after the initial assembly of monomeric silicatein, filamentous structures are formed as a consequence of protein-protein interaction/assembly.[40] (Figure 3)

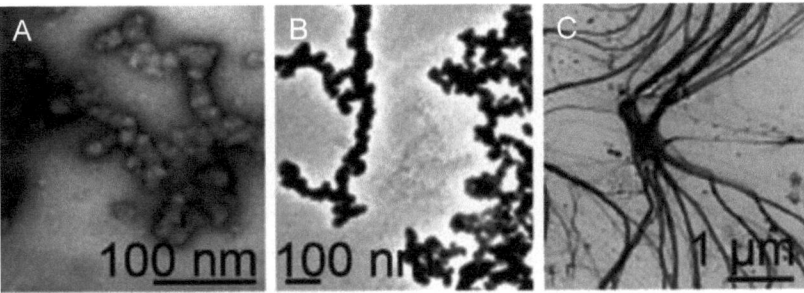

Figure 3. Oligo-/polymerization of silicatein. Silicatein was prepared from spicules (*S. domuncula*) and was then allowed to reassemble in a glycerol-free buffer. After incubation periods of 30 (**A**), 180 (**B**), or 360 min (**C**), samples were taken and analyzed by TEM.

2.3.2.4. Spiculogenesis

Deeper studies on the cellular level of spicule biogenesis (e.g. spiculogenesis) became possible after introduction of a sponge cell culture system – primmorphs.[9,41,42] The process of spicule formation can be divided into an initial intracellular step and a subsequent extracellular shaping phase.

(i)   *Intracellular phase (initial growth):* It could be demonstrated that silicic acid is actively taken up by cells [sclerocytes] via the Na^+/HCO_3-$[Si(OH)_4]$ co-transporter.[43] In parallel, mature silicatein is synthesized/processed and subsequently deposited together with silicic acid in special vesicles of the sclerocytes, called silicasomes. Within silicasomes axial filaments are formed around

which silica is subsequently enzymatically deposited. After formation of a first layer (or a few layers) juvenile spicules are released into the extracellular space, where they grow in length and diameter by appositional growth.[9]

Concurrently to the fractal-like silicatein self-assembly theory, it was recently postulated that the smectite-like nanocrystals are involved in the initial assembly of silicatein monomers and formation of the primary axial filaments (<500 nm) which have not yet started to synthesize silica (Figure 4) in a similar way as found for osteogenesis. (*see below*) These smectite crystals with a size range of 30-500 nm could be visualized always inside of specific sponge cells (sclerocytes) and its structure solve by High Resolution Transmission Electron Microscopy (HR-TEM) with automated diffraction tomography.[44] (Figure 5) Interesting to note that those nanocrystals are associated with the axial filament but in transient form. Identical patterns, reminiscent of crystalline structures, have been discovered in hexactinellid spicules, e.g., *Aphrocallistes ramosus*. The existence of intranuclear crystals in the fresh water sponges *Ephydatia muelleri* and *Spongilla lacustris* had already been described as early as 1995.[45]

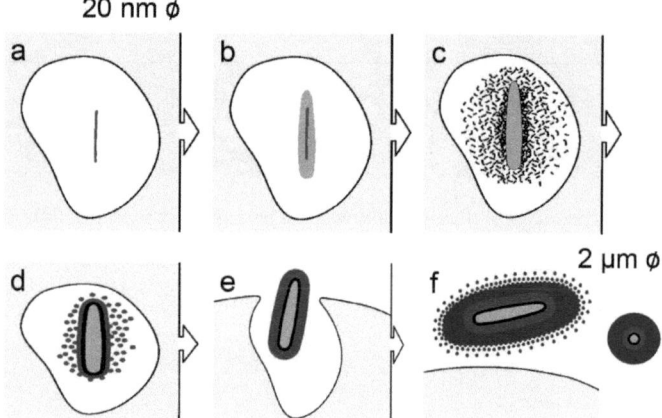

Figure 4. Scheme of spicule development stages; from the initial nanospicule (template) to the released extracellular mature spicule.

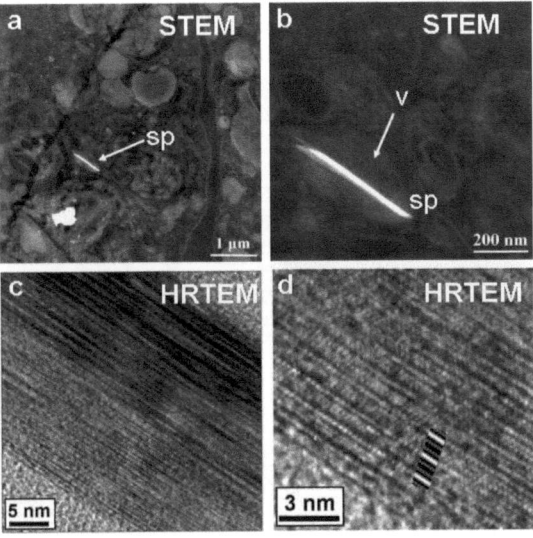

Figure 5. STEM and HRTEM (FFT) analysis of ultra thin stained cuts from primmorphs from *S. domuncula*. (**A**) Overview of a cell (sclerocyte) synthesizing a primordial spicule (sp); (**B**) nanospicule localized intracellularly within a vesicle (v), (**C**), (**D**) HRTEM view down the *b*-axis, with HRTEM image simulated.

(ii)   Extracellular phase - appositional growth/ final morphogenesis: upon spicule extrusion a filamentous strings is created enfolding the newly formed silica structure. These filaments consists of galectin that oligomerizes in the presence of Ca^{2+}, collagen and silicatein (Figure 6A). Interesting to note, that in the extracellular space, silicatein molecules are active and arranged along these filamentous strings.[38] The deposition of silica proceeds over this organic cylinder forming the first siliceous layer. Another organic filamentous layer containing galectin, Ca^{2+}, collagen and extracellular active silicatein, is deposited on the surface of the spicule and again a new silica layer is formed. This process is denominated appositional lamellar growth. In hexactinellids, appositionally layered silica lamellae can reach 1,000 in number.[28] However, spicules growth in 3D, i.e., not only centrifugal growth ("thickening") but also axial growth ("elongation"). It has been demonstrated that accumulation of silicatein at the tip of growing spicules allows the spicules to grow in length.(Figure 6B)

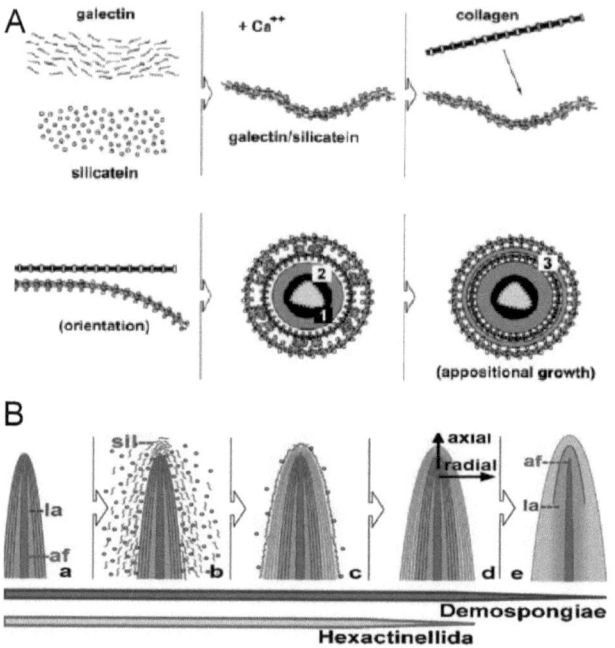

Figure 6. Formation of poriferan siliceous spicules. (**A**) Schematic outline of the appositional growth of spicules from demosponges. (**B**) Schematic outline of radial/axial growth and maturation of spicules during the extracellular stage of spiculogenesis. These siliceous lamellae mostly remain distinct (d; Hexactinellida) or fuse completely by a biosintering process (e; Demospongiae), creating a "solid" siliceous mantel that surrounds the axial filament (af).

So far, the processes described above do not explain the species-specific shaping of spicules, although it has been proposed that spicule shape is depending on the silica availability.[46] This proposed biogenic process is analogous to the one observed during mammalian bone-formation.

Introduction

2.4. Silicatein wide applications

Based on the processes observed during the extracellular growth of spicules (apposition of lamellar silica layers), the natural principle was applied in biomimetic and (nano)biotechnological approaches using Nature as a model. Consequently, the enzymes involved in sponge biosilification, in particular silicatein and silicase, have attracted increasing attention because of their potential applications in the field of nanobiotechnology and biomedicine. Silica-based materials are used in many products including microelectronics, optoelectronics, and catalysts. Biocatalysis of biosilica formation from water-soluble precursors, mediated by silicatein occurs under mild physiological conditions and is advantageous when compared to chemical production methods that require harsh conditions such as high temperatures, pressures or extreme pH.

In the same way as Wöhler (1828) succeeded to synthesize urea from an inorganic material, the enzymatic synthesis of inorganic polymers, mediated by organic molecules, introduced a new framework of research.[47] The following examples show that Nature could be used as a biological blueprint for biomedical and biotechnological applications.

2.4.1. Bionanotechnological applications of silicatein

Silicatein remains functionally active after immobilization of the protein onto metal or metal oxide surfaces.[48] Recombinant silicatein immobilized on a gold surface was able to catalyze the formation of interconnected silica nanospheres with a diameter of about 70–300 nm.[49] The gold surface had been functionalized with nitrilotriacetic acid (NTA) alkanethiol, which binds recombinant His-tagged silicatein through Ni^{2+} complexation whereas binding of nitrilotriacetic acid (NTA) alkanethiol to gold surfaces was also achieved applying the formation of self-assembled monolayers (SAM).[50] (Figure 7A) The range of potential applications of silicatein is increased by the fact that this enzyme is so versatile and is able to catalyze – besides silica (SiO_2) polymers – the formation of other metal oxides like titania (TiO_2), [50,51,52], zirconia (ZrO_2),[50,53] (Figure 7A) and GaOOH/spinel gallium oxide [54] from the respective water-stable precursors at room temperature and neutral pH. These metal oxides are known to exhibit good semiconductor, piezoelectric, dielectric and/or electro-optic properties making them suitable for fabrication of microelectronics, for example, lithography.

Based on these findings, new strategies towards the application of the silica-forming enzymes have been designed. Recently, fabrication of sponge spicule-like core–shell materials (micro level) of alternating metal and metal oxide layers with complex properties was found to be feasible opening a new door to immobilization of silicatein. Layer-by-layer bioinspired nanostructures were recently described with help of a multifunctional polymeric ligand. This multifunctional polymer showed its versatility towards possible functionaliztion of innumerous metal oxide surfaces. It contains dopamine/catechol functional group for attachment of the polymer to the metal oxide surface and NTA chelating molecule for binding of the His-tagged silicatein. For example, His-tagged silicatein immobilized onto polymer functionalized TiO_2 nanowires produced gold nanoparticles on their surface in the presence of tetrachloroaurate anions ($AuCl_4$) by exhibiting a reductive activity.[55] (Figure 7B) Similar examples, were recently described. His-tagged silicatein was immobilized on the surface of γ-Fe_2O_3 supermagnetic nanoparticles (10nm), using multifunctional polymer, resulted in a smooth biosilica coating over γ-Fe_2O_3 nanostructures.[56] (Figure 7C) WS_2 chalcogenide nanotubes functionalized with scorpionate like-polymer and His-tagged silicatein when incubated with titanium alkoxide lead to the formation of layered WS_2-biotitania.[57] (Figure 7 D). Curiously, silicatein has also been shown to catalyze the (ring-opening) polymerization of (cyclic) L-lactide to the biocompatible and biodegradable polymer poly-L-lactide, which is used as a scaffold in tissue engineering. [*see below*, 58]

It has been recently reported that sponge cells – primmorphs – can be used as nano-factories for biological controlled fabrication of hybrid nanostructures. When titanium alkoxide precursor was co-incubated with primmorphs, the presence of this compound did not only it induced cell proliferation and silicatein up-regulation but also lead to the intracellular formation of hybrid materials composed of SiO_2/TiO_2.[59]

Introduction

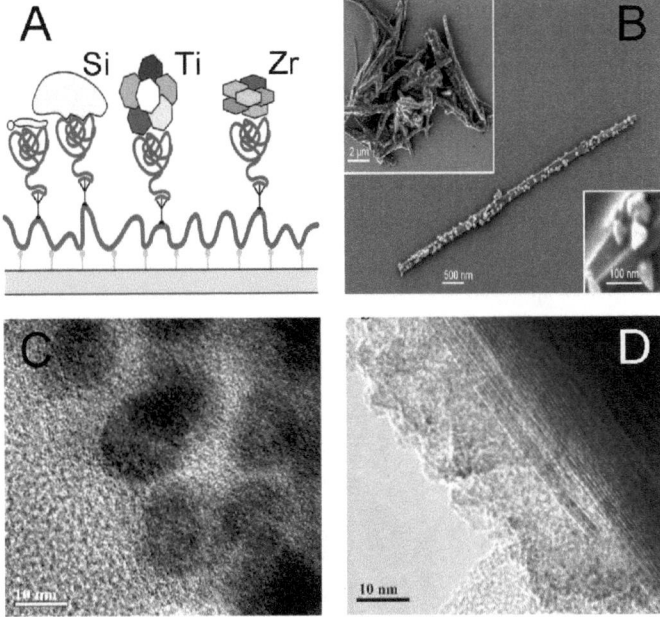

Figure 7. Nanobiotechnological applications of silicatein. (**A**) Recombinant silicatein immobilized on a gold surface functionalized with nitrilotriacetic acid (NTA) alkanethiol. (**B**) His-tagged silicatein was immobilized on polymer functionalized TiO_2 nanowires produces gold nanoparticles due to an reductive activity. (**C**) His-tagged silicatein was immobilized on the surface of $\gamma-Fe_2O_3$ supermagnetic nanoparticles (10nm) using multifunctional polymer forming core-shell Fe_2O_3@biosilica nanostructures. (**D**) WS_2 chalcogenide nanotubes functionalized with scorpionate like-polymer and His-tagged silicatein and incubated with titanium alkoxide lead to the formation of layered WS_2-biotitania.

2.4.2. Biomedical approach

Silica is an essential nutrient for the natural ecosystem in general [60] and for humans and other low ertebrates in particular [61,62] where silicon deprivation results in severe skeletal malformations.[63] Moreover, a spatial correlation could be established between the areas of bone formation within animal tissue and the accumulation of silicon. Thus, a burst of silicon accumulation was seen around the osteoid and osteoid-bone interfaces, suggesting that this inorganic component is essential for bone formation. (Figure 8A) Consequently, the effect of silica, enzymatically catalyzed by silicatein, on the activity of osteoblasts was investigated in depth. Indeed, the cell model used (human osteogenic sarcoma cells; SaOS-2) displayed an increased mineralization activity, when cultivated on biosilica surfaces.[64] In particular, coating of the substratum with biosilica and type 1 collagen not only increased the cellular Ca-phosphate deposition but also stimulated cell proliferation. (Figure 8B) In subsequent studies the effect of biosilica and silica-based components on the expression of key genes involved in formation of tooth enamel - amelogenin, ameloblastin, and enamelin – was investigated. These studies revealed that the combination of ß-glycerophosphate and silica-based components increased the expression of these marker genes (Figure 8C) and was further supported by the increased deposition of hydroxyapatite crystallites on the surfaces of these cells.[65] (Figure 8D)

First attempts to evaluate the biomedical application of silicatein/biosilica for treatment of bone defects are promising and are described in depth throughout this Ph.D. thesis.

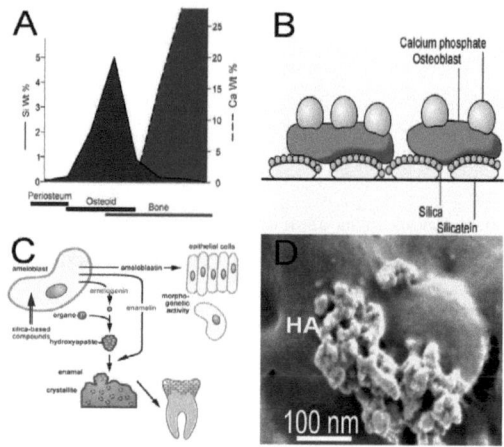

Figure 8. Biomedical application of biosilica and silicatein. (**A**) Temporal relationship between silicon accumulation and calcium composition during early stages of bone formation in rats. (**B**) Schematic representation of the effect of silica-based components on the expression of the three marker genes (amelogenin, ameloblastin, enamelin) in ameloblasts. (**C**) Schematic representation of biosilica and type 1 collagen substratum coating resulting not only increased the cellular Ca-phosphate deposition but also stimulated cell proliferation The silica-based components stimulate the expression of amelogenin, resulting in the formation of nanospherical hydroxyapatite around which hydroxyapatite crystals are deposited. (**D**)

2.5. Calcium Phosphate biominerals

In the field of biomineralization, the phylum Chordata is the most extensively studied. The notion that mineralization on the cordates is synonymous with calcium phosphate is partially true, specially for the mineralized skeletal hard parts of most of Craniata or vertebrates. The calcium phosphate mineral found is partially and variable carbonated, usually, in the form of dahllite.[66,67] Mineralized cartilage is quite different in ultrastructural organization from bone or dentin, even though its major constituents are also collagen fibrils and apatite crystals. Tooth enamel is distinct from bone, dentin and cartilage and its organic phase does not include collagen.

Although this topic has been extensively revised and constantly updated, the following sub-chapters will focus on the biomineralization process of bone as we know it nowadays.

2.5.1. Bone

2.5.1.1. Bone has functional biomineral in animal evolution

Bone is a vascularized, dynamic tissue serving physiological, protective and mechanical functions to the animals. The physiological function of bone includes hematopoiesis (production of red and white blood cells) and mineral homeostasis. In fact, bone can actively work as mineral deposit where various ions such as calcium, potassium, carbonate, magnesium, strontium, chloride or fluoride, can be used without compromising its overall structure or mechanical properties.[68] As a product of biomineralization and evolutionary process, the structure and properties of bone vary according to its location fulfilling the necessary functions. For example, human skeletal elements, such as the skull and scapula (shoulder blade) are not subjected to extensive loading and have a different structure/morphology when compared to long bones, i.e., tibia and femur. The latter ones, resemble a hollow cylinder in an evolutionary optimized design to withstand compressive and bending forces, fracture and fatigue resistance.[69-71] Bone is structurally well ordered with several hierarchical levels that reflects its overall unique properties (Figure 9) and is the final result of several evolutionary readjustments.

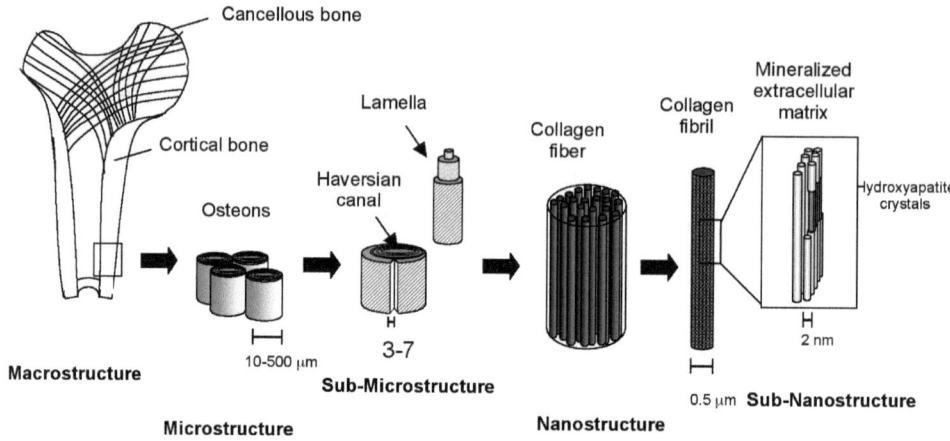

Figure 9. Schematic representation of bone hierarchical structure. Microstructure (cortical bone) consists of osteons with Haversian canals and lamellae. Nanostructure shows collagen fibers structural units surrounded by bundles of mineralized hydroxyapatite crystals.

2.5.1.2. Bone hierarchial composition

Bone is classified as a composite-like tissue and its basic constituents has a high content of heterogeneous carbonated apatite crystals (70% wt) as reinforcement phase embedded in an elastic organic matrix (30% wt), that acts both as 'glue' to hold the mineral phase and secures a proper organized structural arrangement (templating).[72, 73] However, what makes the bone a unique and complex biomineral are its mechanical properties. These depend on several factors such as mineral/organic matrix ratio, porosity, degree of cross-linking and interaction (both physical and chemical) between its constituents.[71, 74] Since its discovery, the collagen present in mineralized bone gives the same characteristic periodic banding pattern as unmineralized bone.[75] It became evident that a close association exists between the crystals and the collagen and this was the key for understanding the molecular organization of bone as the structure of collagen itself.

From the inorganic point of view, the bone is formed by mineralized crystals, identified as calcium phosphate in early 20's, [76, 77] and from that point on is referred as hydroxyapatite ($Ca_{10}(PO_4)_6(OH)_2$). At the nanoscale, hydroxypatite nanocrystals are partially carbonated (4-6%wt) and have an elongated morphology, typically on the order of tens of nanometers in length and several nanometers wide and a preferred crystallographic and morphological orientation along directions of major stress.[69,78] The size of the crystallites is very important for events such as bone repair. The time for formation of small crystals is rather fast consequently leading to a fast mineralization/regeneration process.

Bone organic matrix counterpart is composed (80-90% wt) of biopolymer fibrils, i.e., in its majority collagen (type I), non-collagenous proteins including osteonectin, α2-HS glycoprotein, osteocalcin, bone sialoprotein, and osteopontin as well as small proteoglycans, such as decorin and biglycan.[3] Collagen type I structure is composed of a series of interwoven molecules arranged in a staggered triple helix forming a fiber-like structure with preferential orientation.[79] Although these fibrils can differ in size, the larger collagen fibrils are found to be 15 mm in length and 40–70 nm in diameter. The primary structure of collagen type I was determined, comprising a sequence of about 20 different amino acids. Among the three well-oriented polypeptide amino acid chains, the location of inter- and intra fibrillar cross-linking sites contributed significantly to a deeper comprehension of some bone properties.[80, 81] These cross-linkages between collagen fibrils not only stabilize the complete network providing high tensile strength and stiffness and but can also act as a template. However, collagen *per se* shows low compression or shear properties and thus the presence of a mineral counterpart is essential. Hydroxyapatite crystals are dispersed throughout the matrix in gaps between collagen fibrils. However hydroxyapatite crystals *c*-axis are well perfectly aligned with the collagen fiber axis [82] significantly improving bone mechanical properties by offering higher strength and stiffness under compressive stresses. At the microscale level, bone structure is composed by fundamental units designed as osteons. These consist of concentric lamellae with approximately 3–7 mm in diameter, oriented in the longitudinal direction and well-orientated, and Haversian system or secondary osteons.[83] The Haversian channeling system is formed secondarily, i.e., after initial bone has been laid out and forms canals, with variable pore size (few microns to a couple of hundreds of microns in diameter), that allows supply of blood and nutrients to the tissue.[83] Finally, at the higher organizational level (macroscale level) bone can be differentiated between compact (solid, externally) and cancellous bone (spongy, internally).

2.5.1.2. Bone biomineralization

Bone biomineralization, in its basic features, is very similar to all the other organic matrix-mediated processes already known. However, to compare this process, an understanding of bone formation requires deeper insight on different stages of the overall process.

It was discovered that early stages of many bone and bone-like tissue (cartilage and dentin) do not involve synthesis and extracellular self-assembly of the organic matrix framework (collagen) as previously supposed but instead it comprises initial intracellular mineral formation A representative general bone biomineralization sequence of temporal events can be drawn is described below. (Figure 10)

The early stage of bone mineralization starts with the cellular uptake of ions such as calcium and phosphate (Figure 10A) forming intracellular vesicles (membrane-bound vesicles) highly rich in acidic phospholipids such as phosphotidylserine and phosphotidylinositol.[84, 85] (Figure 10B) The function attributed to these vesicles in bone biomineralization process is a temporary storage site for calcium and phosphate ions in an amorphous form (e.g. amorphous calcium phosphate - ACP), needed for collagen mineralization (Figure 10B). Curiously, the presence of such vesicles was also been reported for other ions and other organisms like, for example, diatoms, chitons and sponges.[3,5,86]

Surprisingly, the amount of intracellular vesicles depends on the age of the animal and is directly correlated with bone regeneration capacity, i.e., the younger the animal, the higher vesicle content and consequently the higher and faster bone regeneration capacity.[85, 87]

In bone intracellular mineral formation, the vesicles are located further away from the mineralization site (Figure 10B) where the somewhat closer vesicles display a templating function that surprisingly contains partially amorphous material proposed to be a transient intermediate in the form of octacalcium phosphate (OCP) from where hydroxyapatite starts to nucleate.[88] (Figure 10C) Close to the mineralization front, the mature vesicles contained exclusively crystalline deposits [85] with needle-like shape composed essentially of hydroxyapatite [89] that are able to rupture the vesicle membrane being released into the extracellular space.[90] This is also referred as mineralized nodules. (Figure 10C) According to this theory, in first stages of bone biomineralization, minerals (transient intermediate OCP and hydroxyapatite) are not closely associated with collagen framework but immediately after its release into the extracellular space, the mineralized crystals are transported to already self-assemble collagen matrix (Figure 10D) and it starts to biomineralize by filling in the gaps (2/3) that previously contained water.[91] (Figure 10E)

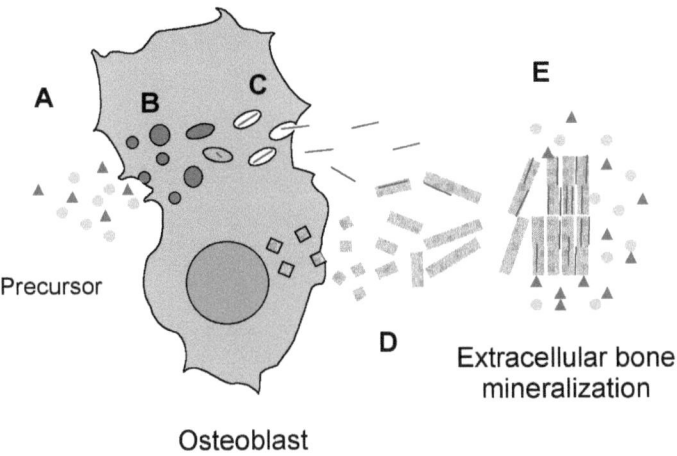

Figure 10. Schematic representation bone biomineralization at different stages.

Another theory, named nucleation (seeding) theory was proposed where crystals nucleate extracelullarly in these holes or even at the surface of the self-assemble collagen matrix.[81] In the 50's a framework for understanding dynamics between extracellular fluid mineral composition and hydroxyapatite crystallization was established. It was discovered that extracellular space has to be supersaturated regarding bone essential ions, i.e., calcium and phosphate in order for the mineralization to occur.[68] The localization and distribution of both ions is well known. Calcium ions are closely localized with proteoglycans and phosphate ions in collagen fibrils. These ionic separations control precisely the production of hydroxyapatite crystal formation by inhibiting uncontrolled precipitation of crystals through a local regulation mechanism. Of course, this is a simplified version that supported nucleation(seeding) theory that nowadays has been proven to be incomplete.

Nevertheless, bone mineralization is a continuous and dynamic process, alike other mineralized tissues, forming in a step further (after collagen mineralization) the Haversian channeling system, for example. Interesting to note that, even during mature stages, the bone is frequently remodeled by cells that are controlled by hormones in order to maintain constant the calcium levels in blood serum.[92]

The cells that constitute bone can be categorized in three types: (i) osteoblasts, which synthesize bone matrix; (ii) osteocytes, cells embedded within bone matrix and (iii) osteoclasts, responsible for bone matrix catabolism. Bone undergoes a continuous cycle remodeling, i.e., bone destruction and reconstruction orchestrated by these cells. Osteoblasts have been by far the most studied cells. Its function is related both with lay down new bone mineral and osteocytes differentiation as a consequence of eventual embedment into the new mineralized matrices. These osteocytes have the function of maintaining the mineralized matrix for a certain period and may also regulate mechanical stress in bone.

The hierarchical composite structure of bone, at the macro-, micro- and nanoscales, is still not completely understood and remains a challenge specially to bone regeneration research field. Although much research has been carried out so far, understanding nanoscale contributions to (i) cell responses and (ii) mechanical properties is still ongoing.

2.6. Tissue engineering

2.6.1. Overview

Tissue engineering is nowadays a major expansion research field and sets its goals in repairing and regenerating damaged human tissue by integrating different disciplines such as engineering, transplantation medicine, and life sciences. The relatively new interdisciplinary field has been rapidly evolving in an attempt to address the increasing needs of rapid bone regeneration within a population with bone fractures and/or defects and reduced regenerative capabilities.

The concept of ideal bone substitute, as been known through many years as the "Holy Grail" of regenerative medicine. This concept idealizes a device that, above all, rely on the same biomineralization process as for the normal bone development. Consequently, it must accomplish a great amount of requirements, such as, it must sustain and promote cellular functions including cell adhesion, proliferation, migration, and differentiation. It should also promote tissue in-growth and development and possess adequate mechanical properties throughout intrinsic remodeling properties and resorption (biodegradable) by the body without adverse biological reactions (e.g., inflammation or an allergic reaction) leading to a *restitutio ad integrum* of the bone defect.

Traditional approaches are distinctly classified as either (i) biological/medical, where bone graft plays a major role; or (ii) synthetic and/or biomimetic. Unfortunately, from the experimental results achieved for many years of bone regeneration research it is now well known that the traditional approaches are still far from the concept of an ideal bone substitute.

2.6.2. Biological/medical approach

2.6.2.1. *Bone grafts*

The most straightforward approach used for bone defects and non-unions caused by trauma, tumor resection, pathological degeneration, or congenital deformities have been traditionally repaired by using explanted bone from a donor site and re-implanted into the defected site. This approach is called *bone graft*. According to a international survey, the average number of bone graft surgeries performed, *per year*, worldwide overcomes two million corresponding to US$2.5 billion.[93] For example, in Germany, 125000 bone grafts are harvested *per year* according to data published at the end of 2008.

Bone graft can be classified into three different implantation processes according to the origin of the explanted bone:

(i) Autografts (autologous) – bone graft is obtained from the patient itself, normally from the iliac crest due to the unavailability of spare bone.

(ii) Heterografts (heterologous) – bone grafts from different donor than the patient itself. Normally these bone grafts are deposited in bone banks.

(iii) Xenografts – Transplantation from an animal of one species to an another, for example from bovine to a different species, normally humans.

Among the above described implantation processes, autograft bone is widely accepted by surgeons, physicians and patients as the most effective grafting material and is still considered as the gold standard in the field of bone reconstruction. Such type of transplant (graft) is very well tolerated after implantation and rapidly integrated with the surrounding tissue as it produces a high bone osteoconductivity, osteoinductivity, and osteogenicity.[94] However, limited amount of spare bone, necessity of performing an additional surgery and rapid resorption of the bone graft (faster than bone regenerative capacity) sets restrictions for application of this clinical process.

Heterografts came along to overcome limited availability requirements of bone and the high clinical demand. Heterografts, although more abundant than autografts, carry a series of limiting factors such as undesired immune reaction, risk of severe and chronic infections and disease transfer. Nevertheless, heterografts are also highly osteoconductive and osteoinductive and constitute a considerable part of clinical pratice since after implantation of artificial devices (e.g., artificial hip joints) the spare bone can be re-implanted.

However, due to the high demand of bone substitutes, the use of heterografts is also not sufficient enough to fulfill the requests. An unlimited supply of bone grafts (xenografts) can be found in other animals, such as cows or pigs. This would be probably the ideal scenery for clinical bone repair. But concerns about immune reactions and risk of disease transfer and infections became more and more highlighted. For example, bovine bone grafts produces high bone conductivity but carries a risk of bovine spongiform encephalopathy (BSE) disease transfer. Therefore, the use of xenografts can only be possible after heat and/or extensive and harsh chemical treatments offering a new bone substitution biomaterial with structural features similar to the natural bone, creating a new opportunity to fulfill the clinical demands associated with an increased economic value. However, this physical and/or chemical treatment of the xenografts renders the material inert from the osteoinductive point of view, loosing its regenerating properties.

2.6.3. Synthetic and biomimetic materials

Material science is a research area that has met a great development in past decades especially in bone substitution materials where materials with a more or less biological relationship have been highlighted as an alternative to bone graft implantation processes.

Bone substitution materials are well known for a long time. It has been reported that the Maya Indians of Honduras used mother of pearl (nacre), around 2000 years ago, as a dental implant with fascinating results.[95] In the early 90's the experiment was repeated yielding unarguable excellent osteointegrating results.[96, 97] However, once more the balance between the clinical demands and the bioavailability limited further use of nacre. Currently, researchers are trying to understand process behind mother of pearl (nacre) biomineralization, in order to replicate structurally mother of pearl through a synthetic approach that can yield, hopefully, also fascinating results.[for a complete overview see ref.98]

The requirements for designing a material that biomimics bone are manifold and so far it was impossible to fulfill all into the same implantable biomaterial. Among these requirements, the material should have sufficient mechanical stability, biodegradability (e.g., to allow bone in growth at the implantation site), high porosity (e.g., interconnected pores to allow cell invasion and nutrients to flow through), absence of components that might provoke cell death and/or immune reaction and their release, possibility of adjust the shape of the implant during surgery according to the patient needs, good sterilizability, storability and processability and a lower price to permit wide clinical application.

A number of synthetic biomaterials that tryto mimic the original bone have been developed and studied both *in vitro* and *in vivo* and some are already available in the market. These new biomaterials include ceramics, sintered ceramics, bone cements, polymers, metals, composite, bone substitutes of biological origin and biofunctionalized materials.[99] However, due to the vast existent literature only some examples will be given.[99]

Ceramics such as calcium phosphates, which exist in a different chemical structures (hydroxyapatite and β-tricalcium phosphate) and are similar to bone and tooth mineral, have been commonly used due to their biocompatibility.[100] (Figure 11A) However, hydroxyapatite based biomaterials show slow biodegradability (e.g. causing problems if further traumatic factures occur at the same time), difficult to process and an inherent brittleness that lead to mechanical failure. Sintering process was developed to overcome the latter problem originating the so-called sintered ceramics, although body resorption is even lower.[101-104]

Bone cements can work as defect filler or like a "glue" by filling the free space between the material and natural bone and have been used successfully to anchor artificial joints (hip joints, knee joints, shoulder and elbow joints) (Figure 11B) for more than half a century. It can include systems such as (i) free radical polymerization of polymethyl methacrylate (PMMA) (Figure 11B), commercialized under the name of Periglass, (ii) precipitation *in situ* of carbonated apatite [105, 106] and (iii) glass ceramics, known by Bioglass® which are based on "CaO-P_2O_5-SiO_2" with adjustable properties depending on the composition.[107] (Figure 11C)

Polymers offer a wide range of possibilities within bone substitute materials due to higher elasticity, biodegradability and biocompatibility and variable composition (e.g. chain length, crystallinity, co-polymer and/or polymer blends).[108-110] Consequently, it seemed that researchers selection of biomaterials shifted towards biodegradable polymeric scaffolds. However, in this case it must be insured that degradation products monomers or oligomers) do not act as immune activators causing inflammation in the surrounding tissue and, in a acute form, symptoms of infection. On the other hand, polymers such as PMMA and its derivatives are produced by free radical polymerization where not only free radicals are formed as intermediates but also unreacted monomers (known to be highly toxic) are present at the implantation site. Moreover, the heat produced during the polymerization reaction damages the surrounding tissue and curiously, although widely used in clinical pratice, PMMA does not induce bone formation. Polymers such as polyglycolide (PGA) or poly(D,L-lactide) (PLA) and co-polyesters are biodegradable and highly biocompatible and commonly used in bone regenerative medicine as substitutes as well as scaffolds and thus by far the most well studied polymers. [111-114] (Figure 11D) The success met by these polymers are that the products of biodegradation (both monomers and oligomers) are easily metabolized.[115] Nevertheless, the accumulation of degradation products of these polymers can also generate inflammation [116, 117] but

Introduction

addition of basic salts to the material introduces the solution.[118, 119]

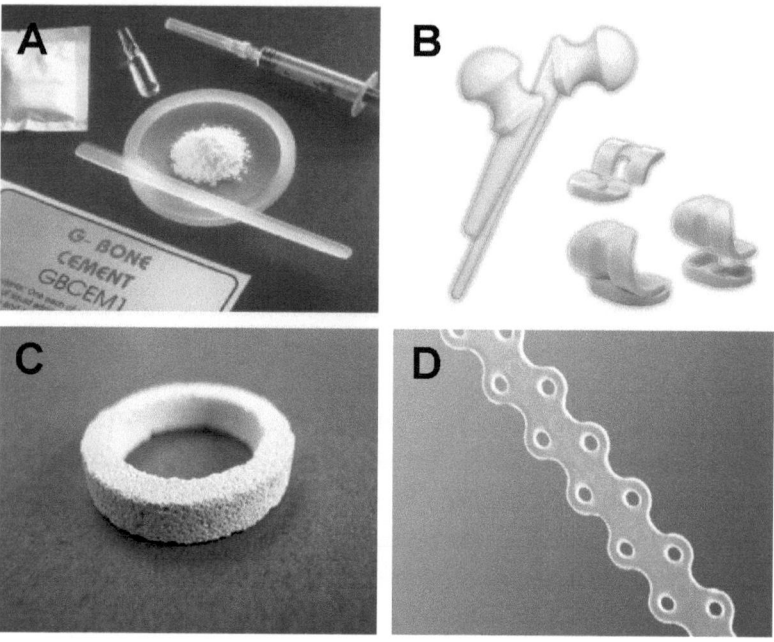

Figure 11. Examples of implants commercially available. (**A**) bone cement composed of hydroxyapatite – G-Bone Cement; (**B**) Hip and knee joint fabricated using polymethylmetacrylate (PMMA) – Hip InterSpace® and Knee InterSpace®; (**C**) Bioglass® ring; (**D**) Poly-DL-Lactide (PLA) bioresorbable bone fracture plate – Zesorb™

2.6.3.1. Silica containing implant: Bioglass®

Among all the materials used for bone substitution, reports using silica are scarce although this element has been shown to enhance osteoblast adhesion, proliferation, differentiation and leading consequently to bone formation.[61] In 1967, L.L. Hench (US Army Medical R&D Command) manufactured a material to fulfill the concept of chemical bond between material and living tissue. Two years later (1969), the same author described the results obtained using a series of silicate glasses that accomplish this goal: formation of bone-material bond![120] These bioglasses were developed within a series of experiments with variable composition of the following major "ingredients": 45-55%SiO_2, 12-24% Na_2O, 12-24% CaO and 3-6% P_2O_5 (% given by weight). The resulting material was generally named bioglasses to signify "special glasses designed to elicit a specific biological response by means of controlled surface reactions."[121]

The exact combination of each element in the overall composition is essential for achieving the desired adhesion exploiting their ability to bond to hard (bone, teeth) and soft (tendons, ligaments) tissues shortly after exposure to the body's physiological environment. Among all bioactive glasses with different compositions, the most investigated was named "45S5", meaning 45% (w/w) of SiO_2 and a 5:1 molar ratio of CaO to P_2O_5 that yielded the best chemical and biological performances.[122] This precise composition was named as Bioglass® has we know it today.[121]

The mechanism of bioactive glasses active remain nowadays inconclusive has it involves a series of physiochemical and ultrastructural events that lead to the formation of a layer of bone-like apatite on the bioactive glass surface within a few hours or days after immersion in a physiological environment. Is this newly formed apatite layer (30 µm) that provides a strong interface bonding between the material and the living tissues. Nevertheless, a commonly accepted mechanism can be assigned. Initially, 9 steps were described [123], where the first 5 steps occur within the first minutes immediately after implantation and the following steps require from 7 to 10 minutes to complete and are the result of the interaction between cells and implant. The 9 steps are described as:

1) Ion rapid exchange between cations (e.g. Na^+ or K^+) present into glass structure with H^+ or H_3O^+ ions from the external solution;
2) Hydrolysis of Si-O-Si bonds, release of soluble silica oligomers and formation of silanols (Si-OH) and monosilic acid ($Si(OH)_4$);
3) Condensation and re-polymerization of SiO_2-rich layer on the surface of the glass inducing changes its morphology forming a porous, gel-like structure;
4) Migration of Ca^{2+} and PO_4^{3-} ions to the SiO_2-surface and interaction via electrostatic interaction;
5) Formation of an amorphous CaO-P_2O_5-rich layer at the surface of the glass;
6) Growth of SiO_2-rich layer (up to 120 µm) by diffusion-controlled alkali ion-exchange; (layer thickness depends on the ratio of Si-glass and alkali and alkaline earth ions)
7) Growth CaO-P_2O_5-rich layer by incorporation of more Ca^{2+} and PO_4^{3-} ions from solution;

8) Crystallization of CaO-P_2O_5-rich layer (up to 30 μm) into hydroxyapatite-like substance with incorporation of OH^-, CO_3^{2-} and F^- ions from the solution;
9) Agglomeration and chemical bonding of apatite crystals around collagen fibrils and other proteins produced by osteoblasts or fibroblasts.

It was previously shown that addition of some multivalent ions such as Al^{3+}, Ta^{5+}, Ti^{4+}, Sb^{3+} or Zr^{4+} inhibit bonding through an unknown mechanism.[124] As for all biomaterials, special attention was addressed to its incredible biocompatibility. Bioglasses safety was tested and showed a remarkable non-toxicity and an excellent biocompatibility.[125] Further experiments (*in vitro* and *in vivo*) carried out by a myriad of independent researchers for several years turned this biomaterial into one of the most successful bioactive materials in clinical use in both surgery and dentistry for more than 30 years.

The fact that Bioglass® (45S5) showed non-toxicity and biocompatibility was discovered later based on studies carried out on surface morphology (porosity) as well as on its chemical structure (amorphous). It was shown by ^{29}Si and ^{31}P MAS NMR spectroscopy that Bioglass® 45S5 has a Si-Q2 type-structure with a small amount of Q3 and Q0 species for PO_4^{3-} ions indicating that these ions do not form a covalent bond and might be simply adsorbed into Ca-Si structure.[125] After this interesting finding, a new question arose and researchers are currently trying to comprehend structure-bioactivity relationships based on accurate structural and chemical data from Bioglass®. The disordered and multicomponent nature of these materials hinders the application of standard experimental probes to access their structure, with the result that prediction and test of compositional effects mostly relies on inefficient and expensive trial-and-error approaches.

3. Experimental Procedure

3.1. Component A: Microencapsulation of silicatein and respective precursor into poly(D,L-lactide) biodegradable microspheres

3.1.1. Production of polymeric spheres containing both silicatein and silica

Poly(D,L-lactide) (PLA) biodegradable polymeric microspheres were fabricated in order to encapsulate recombinant silicatein with the respective precursor (sodium metasilicate). In brief, 1 mL of recombinant silicatein (62 µg/mL) in refolding buffer (1xPBS pH 7.4, 300 mM NaCl, 7% glycerol and 5 mM EDTA) was mixed with a solution of polyvinylpyrrolidone (0.5% (w/v), 5 mg/mL) (P-5288, Avg Mol. Wt.: 360000, Sigma, Steinheim, Germany) for pre-emulsifying the protein. Then, 100 µM of sodium metasilicate (SM) (S-3514, Sigma, Steinheim, Germany) were added to the mixture. Afterwards, the suspension was added into a poly(D,L-lactide) (P1691, Sigma Steinheim, Germany) solution dissolved in methylene chloride (Cat. No. 32211, >99.0% pur., Riedel-de Haën, Sigma-Aldrich, Seelze, Germany) at 10% (w/v) to generate microspheres. The solution was slowly poured into a polyvinylpyrrolidone (PVP) solution (0.5% (w/v)) used as stabilizer, avoiding the common use of detergents. The system was maintained for 6 hrs hours at room temperature under magnetic stirring, in order to let the organic solvent evaporate. The polymeric microspheres were collected by centrifugation (2000xrpm, 10 minutes, room temperature) and washed extensively with distilled water to remove the remaining solvent and stabilizer. The microspheres were freeze-dried using a lyophilizer overnight and termed Poly(D,L-lactide)-silicatein-silica-containing-microspheres [PLASSM]. As control, PLA spheres were produced following the same procedure but in the absence of protein (silicatein).

3.1.2. Physical characterization of PLA microspheres

3.1.2.1. Microscopic analysis of the PLA-silicatein microspheres

The PLASSM were mounted on stubs (carbon adhesive Leit-Tabs No.: G 3347 [Plano, Wetzlar; Germany]) and analyzed by Scanning Electron Microscopy (SEM) (Nova 600 Nanolab; FEI, Eindhoven; The Netherlands) operating at 0.5 kV.

3.1.2.2. Dynamic Light Scattering (DLS)

The PLASSM were ressuspend in phosphate buffered solution (pH 7.2) its dynamic radius determined by photon correlation spectroscopy (dynamic light scattering) using a Zetasizer 3000 (Malvern Instruments, Southborough, Massachusetts, USA) in the 'automatic' analysis mode. The samples were analyzed in triplicate statistically evaluated using the paired Student's *t*-test.[127]

3.1.3. Immunodetection of encapsulated silicatein

3.1.3.1. Immunoblotting

The incorporation of silicatein into PLA microspheres was determined using dot blot technique. PLASSM were dissolved in methylene chloride and sonicated (Ultrasonication water bath, Bandelin Sonorex RK100, Bender&Hobein, München, Germany) for 1 min, until complete degradation of the polymeric shell, and the supernatant analyzed spotted onto a PDFV membrane. As positive control, recombinant silicatein (62 µg/mL) was added drop wise to the activated PDFV membrane and as negative control, poly(D,L-lactide) microspheres (prepared without silicatein) were also spotted after dissolution in methylene chloride and sonication (1 min). The membrane was further blocked in 1% (v/v) blocking solution (Cat. No. 11 921 673 001, Western Blocking reagent, Roche Applied Sciences, Mannheim, Germany) prepared in TBS buffer (10 mM Tris/HCl, pH 8.0, 150 mM NaCl) for 1hr at room temperature in order to block non-specific binding sites. After washing trice with TBS-T (10 mM Tris/HCl, pH 8.0, 150 mM NaCl, 0.05% Tween®-20) for 5 minutes, primary anti-silicatein polyclonal antibody PoAb-aSILIC (1:1000 dilution) in a 1% (v/v) blocking solution (prepared in TBS) for 1 hr at room temperature was added.[9] Afterwards, unbounded primary antibody was removed by washing the membrane trice with TBS-T for 5 min. Subsequently, anti-rabbit IgG-Alkaline Phosphatase-whole molecule produced in goat (1:2000 dilution in 1% v/v blocking solution) was incubated for 1hr at room temperature to form the immunocomplexes. The membrane was than washed trice with TBS-T for 5 min, followed by washing trice with TBS for 5 min and finally equilibrated for 10 min with P3 buffer (100 mM Tris-HCl, pH 9.5, 100 mM NaCl). The immunocomplexes were visualized with the color develop system NBT/BCIP (*p*-nitrotetrazolium blue/5-Bromo-4-chloro-3-indolylphosphate) (4421.1, >98% p.a./A155.1; >99%; Carl Roth GmbH&Co, Karlsruhe, Germany) prepared in P3 solution. The encapsulation yield was determined from averaged triplicate measurements using Quantity One software (v 4.2.9., Bio-Rad, München, Germany) and the results were statistically evaluated using the paired Student's *t*-test.[127]

3.1.3.2. Immunochemistry

In order to verify the effective encapsulation of recombinant silicatein, the PLASSM were subjected to an additional immunochemistry treatment. Two sets of experiments were carried out. On the first set, the microspheres were embedded in glue (UHU plus sofortfest, UHU GmbH & Co. KG, Bühl/Baden, Germany) dried overnight and cut into 50 μm slices using a microtome (Reichert-Jung 2040, Leica Mycrosystems, Nussloch, Germany). On the second set of experiments, PLASSM were analyzed by exposing PLASSM to antibody treatment.

In both cases, the samples were incubated with 1% (v/v) blocking solution (Cat. No. 11 921 673 001, Western Blocking reagent, Roche Applied Sciences, Mannheim, Germany) prepared in TBS buffer (10 mM Tris/HCl, pH 8.0, 150 mM NaCl) for 1hr at room temperature in order to block non-specific binding sites. Afterwards, primary anti-silicatein polyclonal antibody PoAb-aSILIC (1:1000 dilution) in a 1% (v/v) blocking solution (prepared in TBS) for 1 hr at room temperature was added.[9] After the washing twice with TBS-T (10 mM Tris/HCl, pH 8.0, 150 mM NaCl, 0.05% Tween®-20) using a centrifugation step (5000xrpm, 10 min at +4°C), the secondary antibody Cy-3 was incubated for 1 hr at room temperature. After the TBS-T washing step, the samples were analyzed using an Olympus AHBT3 light microscope, together with an AH3-RFC reflected light fluorescence attachment. As negative control, PLA polymeric spheres (without silicatein) were used.

3.1.4. Elemental detection of encapsulated silica

The PLASSM were mounted on carbon stubs (carbon adhesive Leit-Tabs #G 3347; Plano, Wetzlar, Germany) and quantitative elemental distribution analyses were performed through an EDAX energy dispersive X-ray spectrometer (EDAX Division, Wiesbaden, Germany), coupled to a focused ion beam (FIB)-assisted SEM (Nova 600 Nanolab; FEI, Eindhoven, The Netherlands) at an operating voltage of 15 kV and a beam current of approximately 3.0×10^{-9} A. The analytical system was calibrated using internal standards. Ultimately, the data were analyzed using KEVEX Advanced Imaging software (KEVEX Corporation, Foster City, CA).

3.1.5. Release of silicatein from polymeric microspheres

For studying the controlled released of silicatein from PLASSM, we followed the published protocol by co-incubating the polymeric microspheres with simulated body fluid [SBF].[128, 129] Simulated body fluid was prepared as described elsewhere.[129] Briefly, a solution containing calcium (Ca-solution) was prepared using the following components and respective concentrations: NaCl (135 mM)

(Art.no. 3957, ≥95%, p.a., ACS, ISO, Carl Roth GmbH+Co KG, Karlsruhe, Germany), KCl (3.0 mM) (Art.4936, Merck, Darmstadt, Germany), $CaCl_2$ (2.5 mM) (Art.no. A119.1, ≥94%, entwässert, Carl Roth GmbH+Co KG, Karlsruhe, Germany) and $MgCl_2$ (1.5 mM) (Art.no. A537.1, feinkrist. Ph.Eur., E511, Carl Roth GmbH+Co KG, Karlsruhe, Germany). A parallel solution containing phosphorous ions (P-solution) was also prepared using the following components and correspondent final concentrations: Na_2SO_4 (0.5 mM) (Art.no. P032.1, Ph.Eur., USP, BP, Wasserfrei, Carl Roth GmbH+Co KG, Karlsruhe, Germany), $NaHCO_3$ (4.2 mM) (Art.no. 1.06329.1000, Merck, Darmstadt, Germany) and K_2HPO_4 (1.0 mM) (Art.no. P749.2, ≥99%, p.a., Wasserfrei, Carl Roth GmbH+Co KG, Karlsruhe, Germany). Before use, simulated body fluid (SBF) was freshly prepared by adding Ca-solution and P-solution in a 1:1 ratio.

For the kinetic release experiments, 10 mg of PLASSM were immersed in SBF (1mL) for 15 d at 37°C. Them, the polymeric microspheres were centrifuged (3000xrpm, 10 min, 20°C) and incubating solution was replaced with 1mL of freshly prepared solution at predetermined time points over 15d, i.e., day 3, 9 and 15 and the incubating solution (supernatant) was kept frozen at -20°C until further analysis. At the end of the incubation period (15d), the solutions were analyzed by Enzyme Linked Immunosorbent Assay [ELISA]. As a control, PLASSM (10 mg) were incubated at 37°C with distilled water (1mL) and analyzed in parallel by ELISA. Upon the incubation period (15d at 37°C) (both with distilled water and SBF), the PLA microspheres containing silicatein were collected by centrifugation (3000xrpm, 10 min, RT) mounted on a carbon stub, air-dried and its morphology inspected by Scanning Electron Microscopy (SEM).

3.1.6. Enzyme linked Immunosorbent Assay (ELISA)

Samples were slowly thawed in a controlled manner from –20°C to room temperature. Than, aliquots of 100 µL were incubated into a 96-well plate (# 096474, Nunc Immobilizer™, Nunc™, Roskilde, Denmark) for 1 hr at room temperature and the ELISA performed as described.[130] The samples were prepared in triplicate. After protein coating, the 96-well plate were washed trice with TBS and incubated with polyclonal antibodies anti-PoAb-aSILIC (1:1000 dilution in 1% blocking solution) for 1 hr at room temperature.[9] After washing thrice with TBS, the wells were incubated with polyclonal goat anti-rabbit IgG-Peroxidase conjugated (1:2000 dilution in 1% blocking solution) (Code 111-035-003, Jackson Immunoresearch Labs Inc, Cambridgshire CB7 5UE; UK) for 1 hr at room temperature. The development was performed by adding TMB (SureBlue Reserve ™, Cat. no. 53-00-00, KPL, Gaithersburg, USA) until the reaction turns blue. The reaction was quenched by addition of 1M H_2SO_4

into the wells. The absorbance was measured at 492 nm using a 96 well plate reader (Titertek Multiscan PLUS, MKII, Rheinbach, Germany). The results were statistically evaluated using the paired Student's t-test.[127]

3.1.7. Determination of enzymatic activity

For the determination of enzymatic activity, 10 mg of PLASSM were immersed in SBF (1mL) (*see above*) for 15 d at 37°C. After the incubation period, the particles were centrifuged (3000xrpm, 10 min, 20°C) the enzymatic activity of released silicatein was determined by measuring the amount of polymerized and precipitated silica. The protein concentration was determined by Coomassie blue (Roti®-Quant universal, Cat. No. 0120.2, Carl Roth GmbH&Co, Karlsruhe, Germany). In a typical experiment, 2 μg of protein were incubated with a solution of sodium metasilicate (200 μM, prepared in distilled water). After incubation at room temperature for 120 min, the samples were washed with ethanol and polymerized silica was hydrolyzed with NaOH (1M) for 20 min at RT. The quantification was carried out using the classical molybdate-based assay (Silica test, Prod. No. 1.14410.0001, Merck, Darmstadt, Germany) as described elsewhere.[8, 131, 132] As controls, silicatein and freshly prepared SBF were used in parallel. The experiments were performed in triplicate and were statistically evaluated using the paired Student's t-test. [127]

3.2. Component B: Production of plastic-like filler matrix containing silicic acid (PMSA).

3.2.1. Plastic-like filler matrix containing silicic acid (PMSA)

For production of the plastic-like filler matrix, 0.1 g of polyvinylpyrrolidone (PVP) (P-5288, Avg Mol. Wt.: 360000, Sigma, Steinheim, Germany) and 1g of starch (Art. Nr. 4701.1, Carl Roth GmbH&Co, Karlsruhe, Germany) were mixed with 1mL of water glass (sodium silicate solution, S1773, Sigma, Steinheim, Germany) containing approximately 27% SiO_2. Afterwards, water glass was diluted in HEPES buffer (1M, pH 7.1) (Art. No. 9105.3, PUFFERAN®; ≥99,5%, Carl Roth GmbH&Co, Karlsruhe, Germany) to reach neutral pH (1:10 dilution). The filler matrix was than centrifuged at 5000xrpm, for 5 min at room temperature to remove excess of aqueous solutions. The pellet was collected and mixed with 0.3 g of sodium hydrogen phosphate (Cat. No. 1.06346.1000, Merck, Darmstadt, Germany) and the pH confirmed to be 7. PMAS morphology was characterized by Scanning Electron Microscopy (SEM).

3.2.2. Microscopic analysis of the plastic-like filler matrix (PMSA)

The PMSA was mounted on stubs (carbon adhesive Leit-Tabs No.: G 3347 [Plano, Wetzlar; Germany]) and the morphology analyzed by Scanning Electron Microscopy (SEM).

3.2.3. X-ray diffraction (XRD) of the plastic-like filler matrix (PMSA)

The plastic-like filler matrix was grinded and analyzed by X-ray powder diffraction in $\theta/2\theta$ reflection geometry using Siemens D8 power diffractometer equipped with a position sensitive detector. The data was collected using Cu-Kα radiation at an operating potential of 40 kV and a current of 40 mA.

3.3. Bifunctional 2-component implant

The bifunctional 2-component implant was prepared using both components, plastic-like filler matrix (PMSA) and microspheres containing silicatein and silica (PLASSM), mixed in a ratio 1:100 (w/w) shortly before use. The bifunctional 2-component implant was characterized as follows:

3.3.1. Physical properties of bifunctional 2-component implant

3.3.1.1. Hardness measurements

Hardness measurements were performed using a Durometer Shore A - Hardness-Tester PCE-HT200 (PCE group, Germany). The hardness of the PMSA (0.3 g) containing the PLASSM was determined by the depth of indentation created by using a 430 g of load for 15 seconds, according to the American Society for Testing and Materials (ASTM) D-2240 specification at room temperature (23±2°C).[133] Three measurements were done for 0, 0.5, 1, 3 and 5 hr. Data was statistical analyzed.[127]

3.3.1.2. Bifunctional 2-component implant behavior in simulated body fluid (SBF).

30 mg of bifunctional 2-component implant (PMSA and PLASSM, 1:100) were immersed into simulated body fluid (SBF) (see *above for SBF composition*) for 15 d at 37°C, air-dried and its morphology analyzed by Scanning Electron Microscopy (SEM). For comparison purposes, bifunctional 2-component implant was air-dried and analyzed by SEM.

Experimental Procedure

3.3.1.3. Release/adhesion of silicatein to bifunctional 2-component implant: Immunochemistry.
The release and adhesion of silicatein onto bifunctional 2-component implant was studied. For this purpose, 30 mg bifunctional 2-component implant were immersed into simulated body fluid (SBF) (see *above for SBF composition*) for 15 d at 37°C, air-dried and immunochemistry was performed as earlier described (*vide Immunochemistry*). As negative control, the primary anti-silicatein polyclonal antibody PoAb-aSILIC (1:1000 dilution) was replaced by 1% (v/v) blocking solution (Cat. No. 11 921 673 001, Western Blocking reagent, Roche Applied Sciences, Mannheim, Germany) and incubated in parallel for 1hr at room temperature.[9] After the final washing step, the immunocomplexes carrying a chromophore (Cy-3) were analyzed using an Olympus AHBT3 light microscope, together with an AH3-RFC reflected light fluorescence attachment.

3.3.1.4. Adhesion of silicatein to bifunctional 2-component implant: Fourier Transform Infrared spectroscopy with attenuated total reflection (FT-IR ATR) for protein-surface interaction
Infrared analysis of the surface adsorbed protein after incubating bifunctional 2 component implant in SBF for 15 d at 37°C was performed using a Nicolet Nexus spectrometer fitted with a Golden Gate attenuated total reflection (ATR) accessory (Thermo Nicolet). Spectra were recorded at 4 cm^{-1} resolution, averaging 32 scans. As controls, bifunctional 2-component implant before immersion in SBF and recombinant silicatein were analyzed in parallel both in phosphate buffered solution (1xPBS, pH 7.4). PBS spectrum was measured prior to any measurements and further used as background.

3.3.1.5. Imaging properties of bifunctional 2-component implant.
For clinical applications, the *bifunctional 2-component implant* was also analyzed by computed tomography (CT), micro-computed tomography (μ-CT) and X-rays to evaluate the contrast image.

3.3.2. Cell proliferation assay on bifunctional 2-component implant
To test the toxicity of the 2-component implant *in vitro* experiments were performed using colorimetric MTT (3-(4,5-Dimethylthiazol-2-yl)-2,5-diphenyltetrazolium bromide) assay (Cat. No. M2128, Sigma, Steinheim, Germany). [134] MTT is an assay that measures changes in color by detecting the enzymatic activity towards MTT compound reduction to formazan crystals that are water insoluble and display a purple color. MTT (3-(4,5-Dimethylthiazol-2-yl)-2,5-diphenyltetrazolium bromide is initially yellow and than is metabolically reduced by active cells to form insoluble purple formazan crystals, which are than solubilized by the addition of a detergent or dimethylsulfoxide (DMSO). The

absorbance of this purple solution can be quantified spectrophotometrically indicating the percentage of living cells.

HEK 293 cells (ATCC no, CRL-1573, LGC Standards GmbH, Wesel Germany) were grown in Minimum Essential Medium Eagle (# M0643, Sigma, Steinheim, Germany) supplemented with 10% fetal bovine serum (FBS) (#F6178, Sigma, Steinheim, Germany) and 7WD10 cells (kindly offered) were grown in DMEM Medium (Cat. No. 41965, GIBCO, Invitrogen, Karlsruhe, Germany) supplemented with 10% FCS (Cat. no. 15141-079, GIBCO®, Grand Island, NY, USA).

Cell cultures were routinely grown in 50-cm^2 cell culture flasks and were maintained at 37°C, 5% CO_2 and 95% relative humidity. For the cell proliferation assay, HEK and 7WD10 cells were cultured in 96-wells plate accordingly using cell density of $3.0x10^3$ cells/mL. The cells were than incubated with bifunctional 2-component implant with given concentrations (0.140, 0.350, 0.700 and 1.4 mg) in triplicate for 48 hrs at 37°C, 5% CO_2 and 95% relative humidity. Cells were than incubated with a solution of MTT (5mg/mL prepared in sterile 1xPBS, pH 7.4) for 4 hrs at 37°C, 5% CO_2 and 95% relative humidity. Afterwards, dimethylsulfoxide (DMSO; A994.2, Carl Roth+GmbH, Karlsruhe, Germany) was added to the cell cultures and the dissolution formazan crystals was measured spectrophotometrically at 492 nm using a multi-well plate reader Titertek Multiscan PLUS, MKII, Rheinbach, Germany). The results were statistically evaluated using the paired Student's *t*-test.[127]

3.4. Animal experiments

3.4.1. Surgery and implantation

For surgical purposes, sterilization of the PMSA and the PLASSM was performed using a flow of ethylene oxide passing through the sample for 10 min. Both components were to be mixed short before use (implantation) in a ratio 1:100 building up a bifunctional 2-component implant.

Prior to *in vivo* implantation, *ex vivo* studies were carried out. The bifunctional 2-component implant was inserted onto an artificially created bone defect with 3mm diameter in rabbits femur and further analyzed by µ–CT and CT.

The surgery was performed according to a random plan. (Figure 12) 3 animals (Specific-pathogen-free Rabbits; Charles River-WIGA, Sulzfeld; Germany) were operated under anesthesia. Briefly, the operation consisted in preparing carefully both rabbit femurs, avoiding dilapidation of muscles and tendons. Than, two artificial bone defects of 3 mm diameter were drilled in subcondylic proximal and distal positions of rabbit femur. The two sterile components were mixed accordingly and the defects filled according to a predefined plan. (Figure 12) The inner sutures were sewed with self-

Experimental Procedure

resolvent fibres and skin sutures ditto. After 9 weeks the animals were sacrificed and the femurs removed for analysis. Rabbit femurs fixed in 10% formalin and buffered solution were analyzed by optical observation and computer tomography (CT) to evaluate the degree of bone regeneration.

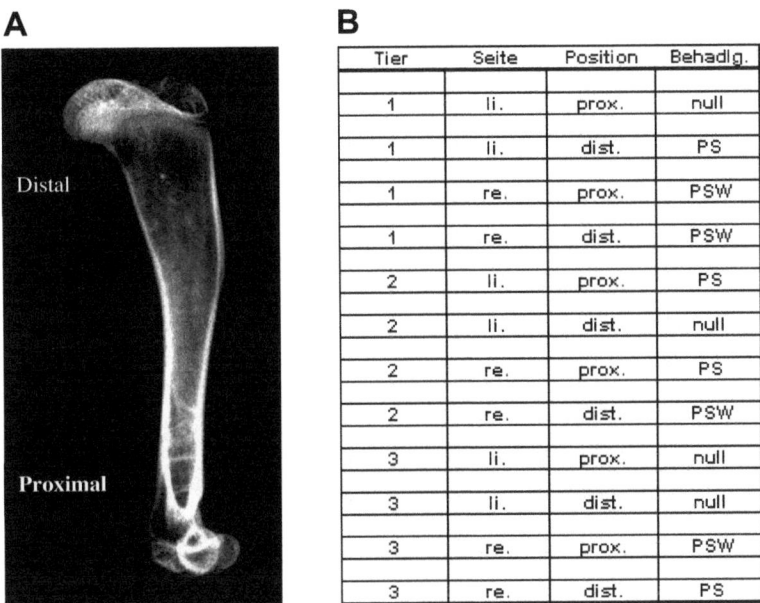

Figure 12. Location of the implants (distal and proximal) on rabbit femurs (**A**). Table of random plan defect filling rabbit femurs and its correspondence with respective animals (**B**). Legend: *Null* - plastic-like filler matrix; *PS* – Poly(D,L-lactide) microspheres containing silicatein and silica; *PSW* – 2-component implant: Poly(D,L-lactide) microspheres containing silicatein and silica and plastic-like filler matrix; *li* – links (left); *re* – rechs (right); *dist.* – distal; *prox.* – proximal.

3.4.2. Computed tomography (CT) and micro-computed tomography (µ-CT) analysis

Computed tomography (CT) imaging of rabbit femurs was done on a clinical 16-slice scanner (Philips Brilliance 16, Philips Healthcare, Germany) with following parameters: tube voltage 120 kV, tube current 300 mAs, detector width 2x0.60 mm, slice thickness 0.65 mm. Femurs containing only the 3mm hole and a similar hole filled with plastic-like filler matrix (*ex vivo*) and after 9 week implantation were examined by a micro-computed tomography system (µ-CT) (SkyScan 1072-100, Aartselaar,

Belgium) using a 100kV X-ray source, equipped with cooled 12 bit grey-scale CCD-camera (resolution: 1024x1024 pixel). The scans performed at 20 μm resolution for 60 min along x axis of the femur set parallel to the plane of the X-ray beam axis.

4. Results

4.1. Component A: Microencapsulation of silicatein and silica precursor (sodium metasilicate) into poly(D,L-lactide) biodegradable microspheres

4.1.1. Production of polymeric spheres containing both silicatein and silica

The aim is to encapsulate simultaneously, the enzyme and its substrate, within the same polymeric compartment using the classical w/o/w methodology with solvent casting. For this purpose, recombinant silicatein prepared in refolding buffer was mixed with polyvinylpyrrolidone (PVP) (0.5% w/v). In this way, protein can be "protected" from direct exposition to organic solvents Sodium metasilicate (SM) in a concentration of 100 µM was added to the polymer-PVP-silicatein mixture. Parallel experiments showed that sodium metasilicate (SM) is not soluble in organic solvents, for example chloroform. In a step further, silicatein-PVP-SM mixture was added drop wise to the solution containing poly(D,L-lactide) (PLA) (10% w/v solubilized in chloroform) to form polymeric microspheres. This step included the use of a brief sonication (10s) that did to disrupt protein 3D structure and consequently its catalytic activity. The second aqueous step in any w/o/w emulsion, involves the addition of a chemical component to stabilize the polymeric microspheres. In the first attempts, a common surfactant (sodium dodecyl sulfate - SDS) was used and its morphology analyzed by Scanning Electron Microscopy.

In a subsequent experiment, PVP was used as stabilizer in order to avoid the use of surfactants due to their cyto- and toxicity. A solution containing PLA microspheres was poured into aqueous solution of PVP (0.5% w/v) and left overnight stirring at room temperature in order to evaporate the solvent. The resulting material was consequently termed as PLASSM, i.e., _PLA_ _S_ilicatein and _S_ilica containing _M_icrospheres. After extensive washing using a centrifugation step, PLASSM morphology was analyzed by scanning electron microscopy (SEM). Figure 13 shows that PLAASM display a non-porous and smooth surface.

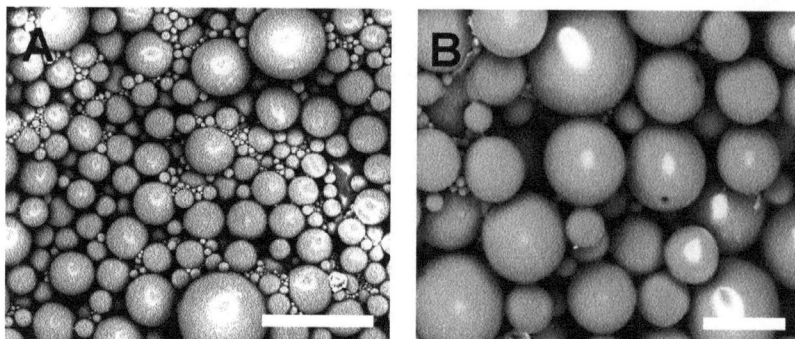

Figure 13. Scanning electron microscope (SEM) images of PLASSM prepared by w/o/w emulsion and stabilized with polyvinylpyrrolidone (PVP; 0.5% w/v) (**A**); at higher magnification (**B**). Scale bar: 1μm.

4.1.2. Physical characterization of PLA microspheres

Morphological analysis of polymeric microspheres stabilized either with PVP (Figure 14A) or surfactant (SDS) (Figure 14B) did not show any significant difference as shown by scanning electron microscopic analysis.

Attempts to study the internal structure (porous or dense) of the PLASSM stabilized with PVP was attempted using atomic bombing, i.e., focus ion beam (FIB). However, this technique is normally used for metallic samples and due to high energy of the atoms bombing (Ge^+), the fragile polymeric/protein sample melted instead of making a straight cut. FIB did not revealed to be a useful technique for internal analysis of PLAASSM.

A study was carried out to determine the size distribution of the PLASSM using dynamic light scattering (DLS). According to the results from DLS analysis (Figure 14C) the distribution size of PLASSM finds two main peaks, indicating a heterogeneous fabrication of microspheres as observed previously by the morphological analysis. After 4 measurements, the average was determined for each of the peaks. The first peak shows a particle size of approximately 1μm with a 10% content in the entire sample. In the second peak there is a higher percentage (90%) of smaller particles, whereas their hydrodynamic radius is of approximately 130 nm.

Results

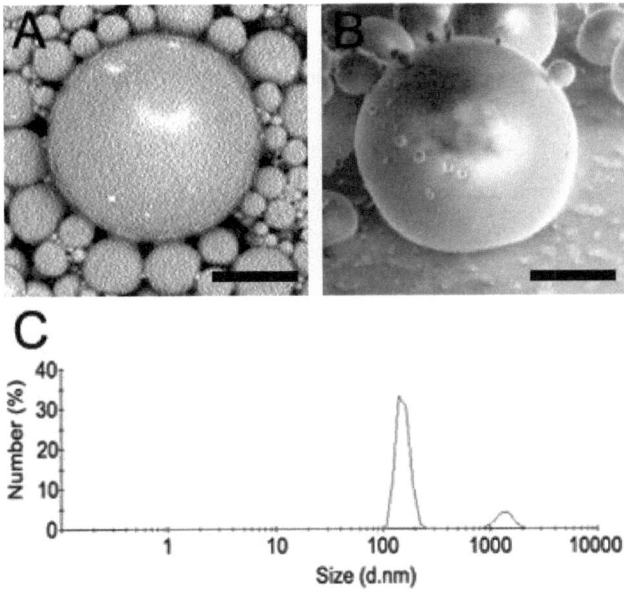

Figure 14. Scanning electron micrographs of PLASSM prepared by w/o/w emulsion and stabilized with (**A**) polyvinylpyrrolidone (PVP) and (**B**) sodium dodecyl sulfate (SDS). Scale bar: 500 nm. (**C**) Dynamic light scattering plot of PLASSM stabilized with polyvinylpyrrolidone (PVP; 0.5% w/v). Data was statistically analyzed.[127]

4.1.3. Immunodetection of encapsulated silicatein

4.1.3.1. Dot-blot

In order to confirm the presence of silicatein into polymeric microspheres an immunobloting analysis (dot blot technique) was performed. (Figure 15) For this metholodogy, PLASSM were re-suspended in methylene chloride, sonicated for 1 min to allow the complete dissolution of the polymeric shell and subsequently release of protein into the medium. Attempts to recover the protein by adding the equivalent amount of water into the extraction vial (containing both PLASSM and methylene chloride) forming a double phase extraction revealed to be unsuccessful. The protein content was measured from the aqueous solution using the classical Coomassie staining procedure. No protein was detected.

However, due to the harsh conditions used (e.g. sonication and methylene chloride) for the release of silicatein from the polymeric microspheres, this has revealed to be only possible way to damage the polymeric encapsulation and consequently no catalytic activity could be measured after protein release.

Nevertheless, after applying this methodology (methylene chloride and sonication), PLASSM supernatant was immediately spotted onto an activated PDVF membrane for antibody treatment analysis. (Figure 15 spot A) As negative control, PLA microspheres that had been prepared using the same methodology as described above, but in the absence of silicatein, were re-suspended in methyl chloride, sonicated for 1 min and spoted onto the same membrane. (Figure 15 spot B) As positive control, recombinant silicatein was used in parallel. (Figure 15 spot C) After solvent evaporation, the PDVF membrane was blocked in 1% (v/v) blocking solution for 1 hr at room temperature, than treated with polyclonal antibodies raised against recombinant silicatein (Poab-aSILIC) for 1hr at room temperature, and finally incubated with the respective conjugated antibody conjugated to alkaline phosphatase.[9] The resulting immunocomplexes were finally visualized using the color develop system NBT/BCIP. As showed in Figure 3, the polyclonal antibodies (Poab-aSILIC) cross-reacted with the positive control (recombinant silicatein) (Figure 15 spot C) as well as with the PLASSM (Figure 15 spot A) giving a positive and clear signal. Interestingly, under the harsh conditions used for the disruption of the PLASSM, the protein might be completely denatured and yet available for detection via antibodies. On the other hand, the same figure shows an expected absence of signal, when only microspheres containing PLA and PVP were used (Figure 15 spot B). Figure 15 spot A shows a certain signal heterogeneity is a consequence of residual PLA/PVP still present in the sample that accordingly does not elicit the same signal with the polyclonal antibody as shown in Figure 15 spot B. However, this result is not conclusive concerning the exact localization of silicatein and therefore further analyses were conducted.

Silicatein encapsulation efficiency was determined by colorimetric densimetry analysis of the dot blot and not by the classical method based on protein recovery after encapsulation and protein content determination using protein Coomassie staining by the reasons stated above. Additionally, the addition of a pre-emulsifying step conditioned the use of this approach for detecting the protein encapsulation efficiency in our multipolymeric system. However, based on the colorimetric densimetry analysis, the silicatein encapsulation efficiency has been determined to be approximately of 40±2 %.

Results

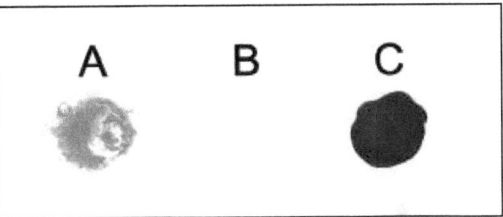

Figure 15. Dot blot analysis of recombinant silicatein encapsulation in PLA polymer re-emulsified with PVP 5% (w/v) and stabilized with PVP (0.5% w/v) solution. PLASSM were re-suspended in methylene chloride, sonicated for 1 min, applied onto the activated PDVF membrane and blocked for 1hr at room temperature with 1% (v/v) blocking solution. After the treatment of the membrane with polyclonal antibodies raised against recombinant silicatein (PoAb-aSILIC) for 1hr at room temperature, an alkaline phosphatase conjugated antibody was added for 1hr at room temperature. The resulting immunocomplexes were finally visualized using the color develop system NBT/BCIP. (**A**) PLASSM shows a clear signal, indicating the presence of silicatein. The heterogeneity of the signal is due to the presence of residual PVA/PVP polymers. (**B**) PLA/PVP microscropheres prepared in the absence of silicatein, show that the antibodies do not cross-react with the single components. (**C**) Recombinant silicatein was applied as positive control and a clear signal is observed.

4.1.3.2. Thin cuts

Immunochemistry in combination with thin cuts was used to determine the exact location of silicatein. For this purpose, two sets of experiments were carried out. In the first set, PLASSM were embedded into a polymeric substrate and air-dried overnight at room temperature. The polymer containing the PLASSM was sliced into 50 μm thin slices using a microtome and treated, first with blocking solution (1% v/v blocking solution, 1 hr at room temperature) to prevent antibodies to react unspecifically with the polymeric surface and then with polyclonal antibodies raised against silicatein (Poab-aSILIC) (1:1000 dilution, 1% v/v blocking solution) for 1 hr at room temperature. Afterwards, the slices were reacted with a conjugated secondary antibody labeled with the chromophore Cy-3. The resulting immunocomplexes were analyzed microscopically. (Figure 16) As control, PLA microspheres prepared in the absence of silicatein were used and the fluorescent images show the complete absence of a fluorescent signal, indicating that the chromophore labeled antibody does not react with the embedding polymeric resin or PLA/PVP blend, thus confirming the previous results obtained with the dot blot technique. (Figure 16A) In contrast, thin cuts of PLASSM treated with Poab-aSILIC, show an intense signal, indicating the presence of silicatein well dispersed within the polymeric spheres confirming the results from dot blot analysis. According to these fluorescent images, silicatein is widely dispersed inside the polymeric spheres. (Figure 16B) However, Figure 16B shows also some agglomerated "free" silicatein that can be attributed to protein release during the immunochemical procedure (e.g. washing steps, antibody incubation). Additionally, from the same image a fluorescencesignal is observed on the background and this not due to unspecific cross-reactivity but it can attribute to thickness of the slices. (Figure 16B)

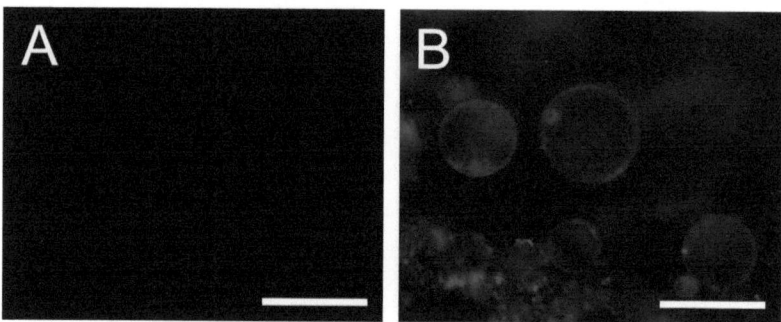

Figure 16. Thin cuts (50 μm) of immobilized PLASSM analyzed by immunostaining, using polyclonal antibodies raised against silicatein (PoAb-aSILIC) (1:1000 dilution, 1% v/v blocking solution, 1hr, RT) to detect the exact localization of protein. The microspheres were then treated with conjugated secondary antibody labeled with a chromophore (Cy-3 labeled anti-rabbit IgG, 1:2000 dilution, 1% v/v blocking solution, 1 hr, RT). (**A**) PLA/PVP microspheres prepared in the absence of silicatein displays no fluorescence signal. (**B**) In contrast, PLASSM shows a clear signal inside the polymeric microspheres, demonstrating the presence of well dispersed silicatein inside the compartment. Scale bar: 1μm

The second set of experiments was carried out to examine the possibility of silicatein adsorption at the outer surface of the polymeric microspheres during the double emulsion process (w/o/w) and solvent casting. PLASSM were re-suspended in a phosphate buffered solution (PBS, pH 7.4). Then, the surface of the microspheres was blocked (1% v/v blocking solution, 1 hr at room temperature) in order to prevent antibodies to react unspecifically with the surface. After extensive washing using a centrifugation step (3000xrpm, 10 min, RT), PoAb-aSILIC were incubated for 1 hr at room temperature (1:1000 dilution, 1% v/v blocking solution). After removing the primary antibodies through extensive washing, PLASSM- PoAb-aSILIC complex were incubated with Cy-3 labeled secondary antibodies for 1 hr at room temperature. (Figure 17A) As control, PLA/PVP microspheres prepared in the absence of silicatein were used and treated under the same procedure. (Figure 17B)

In both cases the absence of fluorescent signals suggests no cross-reactivity between the antibodies and the PLASSM microsphere surface, confirming the previous sets of experiments that: (i) silicatein in not located on PLA-microspheres surfaces after encapsulation; (ii) the PLASSM polymeric blend found at the surface does not cross-reacts unspecifically with PoAb-aSILIC and (iii) that the polymeric microspheres are not porous, since otherwise a fluorescent signal would have been observed.

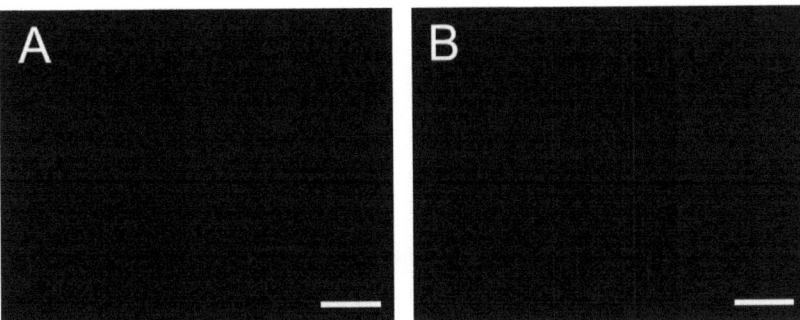

Figure 17. PLASSM immunostaining surface analysis for verifying the possibility of protein surface adsorption during the encapsulation process. The microspheres were successively treated with polyclonal antibodies raised against silicatein (PoAb-aSILIC) (1:1000 dilution, 1% v/v blocking solution, 1hr, RT) and Cy-3 labeled secondary antibody (anti-rabbit IgG, 1:2000 dilution, 1% v/v blocking solution, 1 hr, RT). (**A**) PLA-PVP microspheres (without silicatein) were used as control showing the absence of fluorescent signals indicating that there is not cross-reactivity between the surface of the PLA microspheres and the antibodies (**B**) PLASSM fluorescent image were no signal is observed, indicating that silicatein is not adsorbed at the surface of polymeric microspheres. Scale bar: 50µm

4.1.4. Detection of encapsulated silica source

Silicatein mediates the polymerization of silica monomers, such as tetraorthosilicate (TEOS). [8, 49] On the other hand, sodium metasilicate (SM) is water soluble, completely insoluble in methylene chloride, non-toxic and a very likely candidate for natural substrate of silicatein.

To verify the concurrent encapsulation of silicatein and its substrate in PLASSM, the polymeric microspheres were mounted on a carbon stub and analyzed by scanning electron microscopy coupled to electron dispersive X-rays (SEM-EDX) analyzer, which allowed to determine the elemental composition. The EDX spectrum of PLASSM shows the presence of Si as well as C, O, N and Na, confirming the presence of silicon (Si) inside the polymeric microspheres. (Figure 18B) However, it was not possible to determine quantitatively the amount of encapsulated silica.

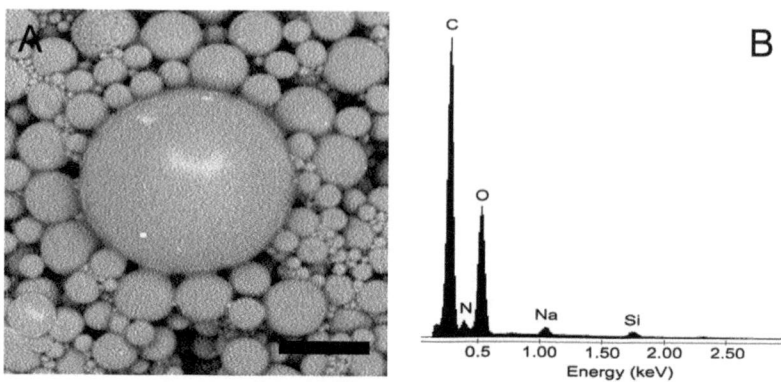

Figure 18. Scanning electron microscopic (SEM) images of PLASSM (**A**) and corresponding energy dispersive X-rays (EDX) spectra (**B**). Silicon signal derived from encapsulated sodium metasilicate (SM) can be clearly visualized in the spectrum. Scale bar: 500 nm.

4.1.5. Release of silicatein from polymeric microspheres

To study the release of the encapsulated enzyme, freshly prepared and dried PLASSM (10 mg) were incubated with simulated body fluid (SBF) in order to mimic the reaction conditions found in the human body. Although there are several variation for composition of simulated body fluid (SBF), we used the 2 component model that involves the mixture in 1:1 ratio of a solution containing exclusively Ca^{2+} cations (Ca-solution) and PO_4^{3-} anions (P-solution) has reported by Kokubo.[129] The samples were incubated for 15 d at 37°C. At day 3, 9 and 15 the samples were centrifuged, the supernatant removed and immediately frozen at −20°C and replaced by newly prepared SBF solution. For comparison purposes, PLASSM (10 mg) were incubated in parallel in distilled water for 15 d at 37°C and analyzed in parallel. The release of silicatein from PLASSM was evaluated by Enzyme Linked Immunosorbent Assay (ELISA) and its morphology analyzed by scanning electron microscopy (SEM).

Figure 19 shows SEM images of PLASSM incubated in distilled water (Figure 19A) and in simulated body fluid (SBF) (Figure 19B) for comparison purposes. Accordingly, after incubation for 15 d in distilled water, the polymeric microspheres retain their round-shape morphology (Figure 19A) whereas after incubation for 15 days in SBF its morphology changed from round-shaped to bulky and unstructured features. (Figure 19B) Additionally, the same image shows still the presence of some spherical microspheres, indicating that polymer degradation, under simulated body environment conditions is an on-going and rather slow process.

The release rate of silicatein from the SSM was assessed by quantitative ELISA technique. (Figure 19C) The polymeric spheres were incubated in SBF medium and in distilled water (control), removed at different time periods (3, 9 and 15d) and assayed in an anti-silicatein antibody-based ELISA. (Figure 19C solid line) The data shows a slow, continuous silicatein release, i.e., after 3 d about 9% of silicatein is released from the SSM, whereas after 15 d the value reaches close to 15%. This value is still far from the 40% encapsulation efficiency previously determined (*see above*). In case of a continuous release under the same rate, the encapsulated silicatein load would be fully released after 40 d of exposure to SFB. (Figure 19C solid line) The data also show that in the control sample, the kinetics of the silicatein release from PLASSM suspended in distilled water is much lower, remaining stable (7%) from the 10th day on due to very slow and constant protein release throughout the polymeric matrix (PVP-PLA-PVP). (Figure 19C dashed line) Consequently, these results show that PLASSM can be kept in an aqueous solution for long term periods of time and demonstrating its suitability for clinical applications.

Results

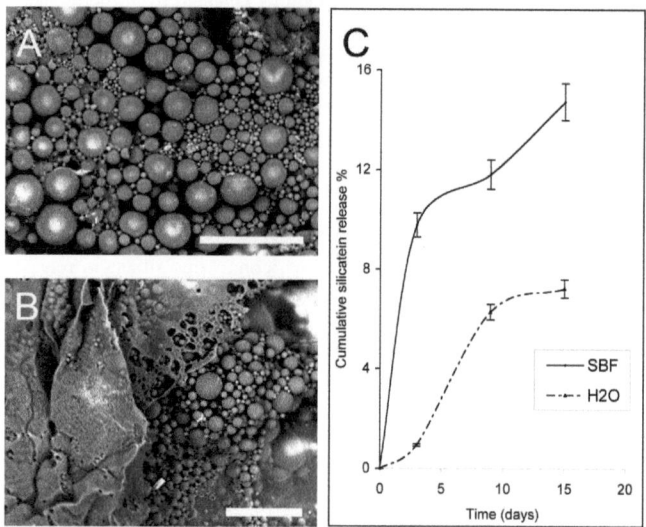

Figure 19. Scanning electron microscope (SEM) images showing PLASSM after incubation for 15 d at 37°C with (**A**) Distilled water and (**B**) Simulated Body Fluid (SBF). Scale bar: 2 µm. (**C**) Enzyme-Linked Immunosorbent Assay (ELISA) plot displaying slow controlled release of silicatein after incubating PLASSM with distilled water (dashed line) and SBF (solid line) for 15 d at 37°C. Data was statistically analyzed.[127]

4.1.6. Determination of enzymatic activity

The catalytic activity of silicatein was determined after incubation of PLASSM in SBF for 15 d at 37°C. Afterwards, PLASSM were centrifuged and the protein content determined by the classical Coomassie blue method. The protein (2µg) was incubated with a solution of sodium metasilicate (200µM) prepared in distilled water and left incubating for 120 min at room temperature. The samples were thoroughly washed with ethanol and the polymerized silica was further hydrolyzed using NaOH for 20 min. Silica polymerization quantification was determined by the classical molybdate assay. As positive control, the same amount of silicatein (2µg) was incubated in parallel and as negative controls freshly prepared SBF (1:1 ratio) was used in parallel.

From Figure 20, the relative activity is depicted taking in consideration the full enzymatic activity as 100% from the non-encapsulated protein for comparison purposes. Upon the release of silicatein onto the "*extramicrosphere*" environment in the presence of SBF, silicatein's catalytic activity is reduced about 25% when compared with its initial activity. From the plot, it can be observed that SBF does not show any activity towards silica polymerization.

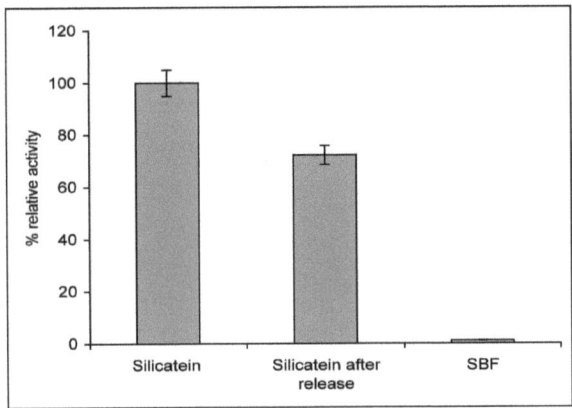

Figure 20. Relative silicatein activity determination upon PLASSM release. The PLASSM were incubated with SBF for 15 d at 37°C and the catalytic activity of silicatein towards sodium metasilicate (SM) was determined based on the amount of polymerized silica by using the classical molybdate assay. As controls, free silicatein (positive) and SBF (negative) were used in parallel.

4.2. Component B: Production of plastic-like filler matrix containing silicic acid (PMSA)

4.2.1. Preparation of a plastic-like filler matrix containing silicic acid (PMSA)

Several ratios of the 4 components (silicic acid, starch, PVP and hydrogenphosphate) were tested. Here the best combination found is shown and proceeded with. In a typical experiment, the plastic-like filler matrix was produced as follows: 0.1 g of PVP and 1g of starch were mixed with 1mL water glass (sodium silicate solution) containing approximately 27% SiO_2. Afterwards, water glass was diluted in HEPES buffer (1M, pH 7.1) (1:10) to reach neutral pH. The filler matrix was then centrifuged at 5000xrpm, for 5 min at room temperature to remove excess of HEPES and unprecipitated water glass. Time-course studies revealed that the precipitated water glass slowly leaches silica monomers/oligomers consequently increasing the pH (around 9 within 2 weeks).

In order to overcome this leaching process with rising pH, which is undesirable for medical applications, the collected pellet was mixed with 0.3 g of sodium hydrogen phosphate and the pH confirmed to be 7. The addition of NaH_2PO_4 compound allows the pH to be stable for at least 2 weeks. Subsequently, PMSA was air-dried at room temperature, mounted on a carbon stub and its morphology characterized by SEM. (Figure 21A) Under these precipitating conditions (1M HEPES buffer) silica particles are formed contrary to the simple precipition in the absence of polymers and display faced-shape and micrometer size (~10 μm). (Figure 21A) Figure 25A shows SEM image of the bifunctional 2-component implant, in which, the polymer (white) that cross-links the silica amorphous particles. Additionally, X-ray diffraction (XRD) analysis of the PMSA revealed its amorphous structure by the absence of define peaks in the XRD spectrum, making this material suitable for biomedical applications. (Figure 21B)

Moreover, combination of these 3 compounds (amorphous silica particles, PVP and starch) with the adjusted ratios allows the formation of a moldable supportive matrix that self-hardens with an adjustable hardening time suitable to be used in an unexpected situation faced by the physician at the moment of the surgery. (Figure 21C)

Figure 21 D to F shows the hardening effect as function of time upon PMSA air-exposure with a certain compositional ratio (amorphous silica particles, PVP and starch). (*see experimental procedure*) Initially, the material is completely soft and easy moldable. (Figure 21D) After 30 minutes, the material has sufficient consistency and hardness to be implanted (Figure 21E), whereas after 3hrs the material loses completely its moldable capacities. (Figure 21F) In this study, the amount of polymers (PVP and starch) was calculated on basis of a medical applicability (surgeon experience), where 15-30 minutes are the required between creating an artificial bone defect in the femur and insertion of the implant material.

Results

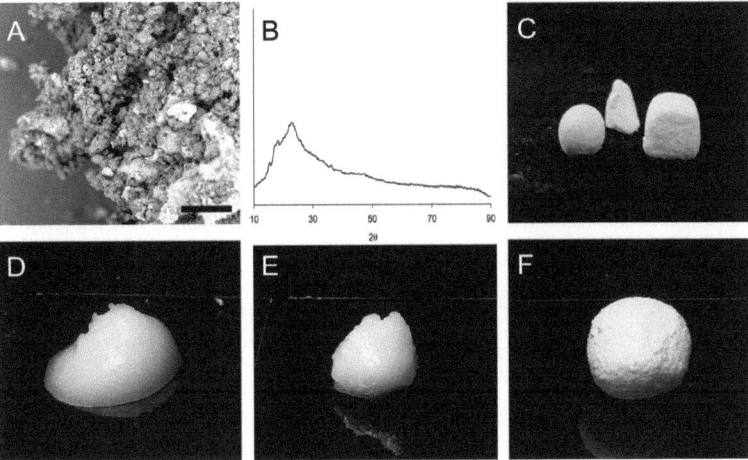

Figure 21. Preparation of a plastic-like filler matrix containing silica amorphous particles (PMSA). Scanning Electron Microscopy (SEM) image of the plastic-like filler matrix. (**A**) Scale bar: 40 μm. XRD pattern of PMSA showing absence of peaks, i.e., an amorphous structure. (**B**) Digital micrographs of the different possibilities for matrix shaping. (**C**) Plastic-like filler matrix (PMSA) at different drying time periods 0 hrs (**D**) 0.5 hr (**E**) and 3 hr (**F**).

4.3. Bifunctional 2-component implant

The bifunctional 2-component implant was prepared using 2 components: (i) PLASSM that contains the active deliverable compound and (ii) moldable (than hard) solid support – PMSA. In a typical experiment, both components were mixed in a ratio 1:100 (w/w) and used throughout all the experiments unless otherwise stated.

4.3.1. Physical properties of bifunctional 2-component implant: Hardness measurements

One of the physical properties required by a moldable 2-component implant is the time during which its hardening takes place. Bearing in mind that, from the point of view of both physician and patient, time is essential and the implant hardening has to be as fast as possible (and required) during the surgical procedure.

Results

Figure 22 shows the hardness kinetics measurements using a Durometer Shore A - Hardness-Tester PCE-HT200 (PCE group, Germany). The hardness of the bifunctional 2-component implant (0.3g) (containing PLASSM and PMSA) was determined by the depth of indentation created on the implant by using a 430 g load for 15 seconds at room temperature (23±2°C), as specified by the American Society for Testing and Materials (ASTM).[133] Three measurements were done for 0, 0.5, 1, 3 and 5 hr, averaged statistically analyzed.

During 0-30 min time frame, the bifunctional 2-component implant transforms from its initial paste-like state to a semi-hard state, making it possible (within this time period) to mold it according to the desired shape. This is considered the ideal time in terms of surgical applications. In the subsequent hours, the implant becomes extremely hard (comparable to a metal surface) with no significant changes in the hardness values after 3 hr. As it can be drawn from the plot, a 2-fold increase on the hardening rate occurs every 30 min and it is plausible to say that the hardening of the bifunctional 2-component implant is a controllable process. (Figure 22)

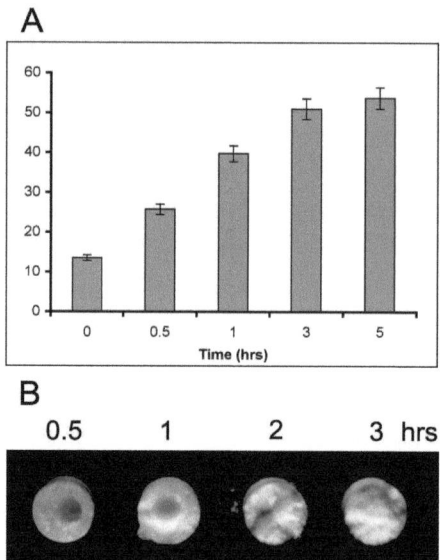

Figure 22. Hardening kinetics of bifunctional 2-component implant using a Durometer Shore A (**A**) plot (**B**) image of indentation. Between 0 and 1hr a 2-fold increased hardening occurs making it suitable for molding and further implantation. After 3 and 5hrs no significant indentation can be visualized and the material loses its moldable capacity. Data was statistically analyzed according to [127].

Results

4.3.2. Bifunctional 2-component implant in simulated body fluid (SBF)

During silica precipitation (PMSA formation) the presence of cross-linking biodegradable and biocompatible polymers (PVP and starch) leads to the formation the silica amorphous microparticles. However, it is difficult to distinguish between these former ones and the PLASSM due to the lack of size differences. SEM imaging of the bifunctional 2-component implant displays unordered packing of these amorphous silica particles and PLASSM and consequently the presence of tiny channels. (Figure 23A) A complementary set of experiments was conducted to study under biomimic conditions, i.e., the properties of the bifunctional 2-component implant were studied in the presence of simulated body fluid (SBF). Accordingly, the bifunctional 2-component implant was incubated for 15 d at 37°C in SBF. Figure 23B shows microscopic analysis of bifunctional 2-component implant after the incubation period. Interestingly, PMSA composite particles are fused forming a highly porous material when compared with its initial structure. Moreover, Figure 23B inset shows an opened PLA-microsphere, located at the surface of the bifunctional 2-component implant, confirming the results obtained for the PLASSM release studies in SBF.

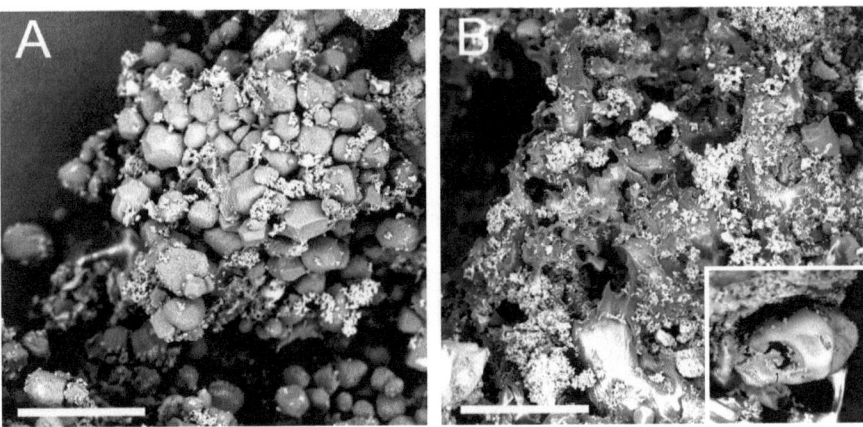

Figure 23. Scanning Electron Microscopy (SEM) images from bifunctional 2-component implant before (**A**) and after exposure to simulated body fluid (SBF) for 15 d at 37°C (**B**). Inset: eroded PLASSM. Scale bar: 30 µm.

4.3.3. Release and adhesion of silicatein onto the bifunctional 2-component implant

In order to co-relate silicatein release from the PLASSM (*see above*) and its possible adhesion onto the slow degrading PMSA, immunochemical and FT-IR ATR studies were performed after the incubation of bifunctional 2-component implant with simulated body fluids (SBF) for 15 d at 37°C. The sample was incubated with a blocking solution (1% v/v for 1hr at RT) to avoid unspecific cross-reactivity between the antibody and the bifunctional 2-component implant components (silica amorphous microsized particles and starch) since it has been previously shown that silicatein polyclonal antibodies do not react with PLA or PVP. (*see above*) Further, polyclonal antibodies raised against silicatein (PoAb-aSILIC) were co-incubated for 1hr at room temperature to the bifunctional 2-component implant. After extensive washing, the implant was treated with Cy-3 labeled secondary antibodies for 1hr at room temperature. As control, the primary antibody was replaced by blocking solution (1% v/v, 1 hr, RT). The resulting immunocomplexes were observed under epifluorescent microscopy. Figure 24A shows a 3D reconstitution of the fluorescent image of the immunostained bifunctional 2-component implant. A clear signal can be observed widely dispersed throughout the sample whereas in the control experiments no signal is present. Moreover, a fluorescent signal can also be observed, not only at the surface, but also inside the channels of this highly porous material as depicted by the 3D image.

Thus, parallel FT-IR ATR studies were performed to: (i) determine the presence of free/unencapsulated protein at the bifunctional 2-component implant and if so, its interaction with PMSA; and (ii) corroborate previously obtained immunochemical results. FT-IR ATR analysis of the bifunctional 2-component implant before and after incubation with SBF for 15 days at 37°C displays a complex spectrum due to its composition (i.e. PVP, PLA, amorphous silica particles and starch) making peak attribution a difficult task. However, a closer look at the range of protein identifying band (e.g. protein amide I band IR fingerprint: 1600-1700 cm^{-1}) can give some hints.

A typical protein FT-IR spectrum contains peaks derived from amide bonds vibrations, e.g., amide I band centered at ~1600-1700 cm^{-1} is largely due to C=O stretching vibrations. Figure 24B (green line) shows free silicatein spectra prepared in refolded buffered solution with a clear band located at 1640 cm^{-1} that can be attributed to the characteristic C=O stretching bond from amide I band.

Moreover, analysis of the bifunctional 2-component implant before SBF incubation shows some bands within this region with small intensity, for example, the band located at 1650 cm^{-1} can be attributed to OH bending vibration modes that are commonly found in the same region than the amide I band. These hydroxyl groups derive from silanol groups (Si-OH) of amorphous silica microsized particles (PMSA), and/or glycosyl groups of starch. (Figure 24B, blue line) The band located at 1750 cm^{-1} is attributed to stretch vibration mode of ketones localized in a cyclic 5-membered ring. In this case only polyvinylpyrrolidone (PVP) chemical structure matches the spectroscopic data.

When analyzing the bifunctional 2-component implant after SBF incubation for 15 d at 37°C (Figure 24B, pink line) there is a clear and significant difference between both IR spectra, i.e., before and after SBF incubation. A change in the environment of the protein led to a shift of amide I band from 1640 cm^{-1} (silicatein free state) to 1670 cm^{-1}, indicating an interaction between the bifunctional 2-component implant and the protein backbone conformation. Once more these results, confirm the possibility of adsorption of silicatein at the surface of the PMSA upon release has describe above. (*see immunostaining results*) (Figure 24C)

One interesting feature of this spectrum (Figure 11B, pink line) is the presence of two additional bands located at lower wavenumbers, i.e., at 1510 and 1590 cm^{-1}. These bands can be assigned to symmetric and asymmetric stretching vibrations of deprotonated carboxylic acid groups originated from the degradation/hydrolysis of PLASSM.

Results

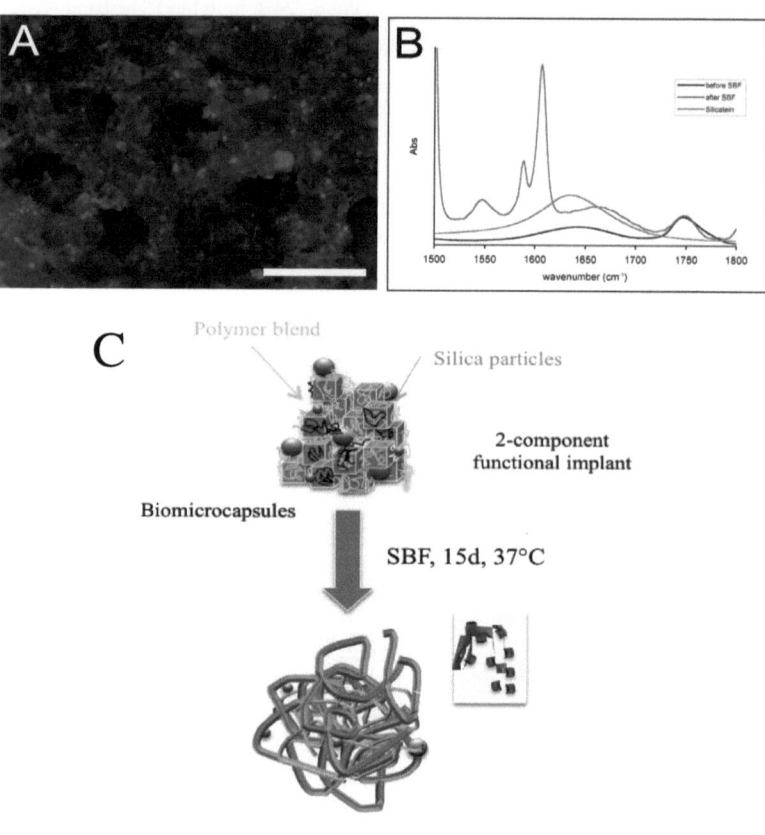

Figure 24. Release and adhesion of silicatein within the bifunctional 2-component implant after incubation with SBF for 15 d at 37°C. (**A**) Immunostaining was performed treating bifunctional 2-component implant with polyclonal antibodies raised against silicatein (PoAb-aSILIC) (1:1000 dilution, 1% v/v blocking solution, 1hr, RT). Then, it was treated with secondary antibody Cy-3 labeled anti-rabbit IgG (1:2000 dilution, 1% v/v blocking solution, 1 hr, RT) to detect the presence of protein adsorbed onto its surface. 3D reconstitution image shows a clear signal throughout the bifunctional 2-component implant indicating adhesion of silicatein onto the PMSA porous structure. (Scale bar: 10 μm). (**B**) Fourier-Transform Infrared (FT-IR) spectroscopy with attenuated total reflectance (ATR) analysis of bifunctional 2-component implant before (blue line) and after SBF incubation (pink line). Recombinant silicatein was used as control (green line). Prior to measurements, FT-IR

Results

spectra of PBS was recorded and used as background. (C) Schematic representation of implant degradation under SFB.

4.3.4. Imaging properties of bifunctional 2-component implant

When considering future medical applications for the evaluation on the degree of bone regeneration without sacrificing the animal or the human, the implant was analyzed, in parallel, by other techniques commonly used in every hospital throughout the world, i.e., X-rays and Computed Tomography (CT). (Figure 25C, D) In both techniques, the bifunctional 2-component implant shows an evident signal, indicating its applicability in regular control of bone growth and development as well as the rate of implant resorption.

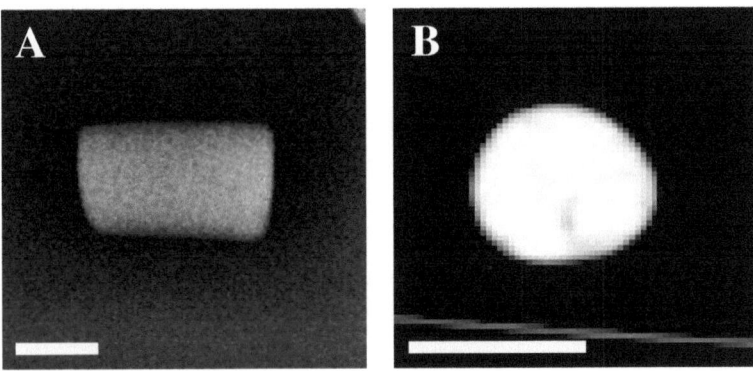

Figure 25. Bifunctional 2-component implant imaging characterized by (**A**) X-rays and (**B**) Computed Tomography (CT). Scale bar: 3mm.

4.3.5. Cytoxicity assay

An important feature, if not the most important one in implant design is the biocompatibility of the putative implant. In order to evaluate biocompatibility of the bifunctional 2-component implant two different cell types were used in combination with the sterilized material. In all sets of experiments, culture medium was supplemented with different concentrations of bifunctional 2-component implant prior to assaying potential cytotoxic effects through a common cell viability test (MTT). The MTT test is based upon the fact that viable cells metabolize (3-(4,5-Dimethylthiazol-2-yl)-2,5-

diphenyltetrazolium bromide (yellow) to formazan (purple) that can be measured spectrophotometrically.

The first cells to be tested were HEK293 cells (human embryonic kidney cells). The HEK 293 cell line was generated by adenovirus transformation and has many properties similar to immature neurons.[136] The use of HEK 293 can give a closer idea about the cytotoxicity in general as well as for under development immature neurons. Figure 26A shows HEK293 cell viability when co-incubated with different concentrations of bifunctional 2-component implant for 48 hr. In the presence of 0.14 mg there is a decrease of 10% in cell viability with an decreasing inverted trend between concentration and cell viability, i.e., the increasing concentration of bifunctional 2-component implant leads to a decrease of cell number. However, at a maximum of 1.4mg tested (10-fold) there is only a decrease in cell viability of 30% when compared with the control indicating that this material is not cytotoxic and be safely used in biomedical applications.

Since not all cell lines react in a similar way exposure to the same molecules, the response of a different cell line [chinese hamster ovary cells (7WD10)] to different concentrations of the bifunctional 2-component implant material was evaluated. Figure 26B shows the relative viability of 7WD10 cells that had been incubated with the bifunctional 2-component implant at different concentrations (0.14, 0.7, and 1.4 mg) for 48hr. In this case, the material, independently from its concentration, shows no cytotoxic effects or significantly inhibition of cell proliferation.

Taken together, the cytotoxicity results obtained for bifunctional 2-component implant indicate that this material and all its components are suitable for further medical applications.

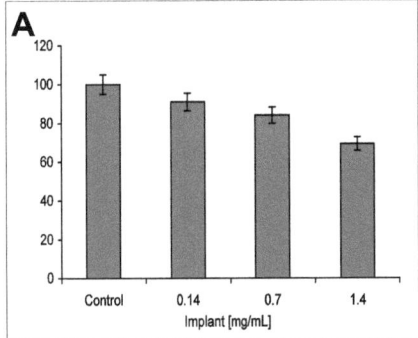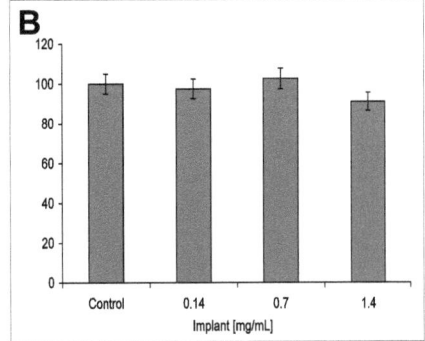

Figure 26. Cell viability assay (MTT) of embryonic kidney cells (HEK293) (**A**) and chinese hamster ovary cells (7WD10) (**B**) to determine the effect of different concentrations of bifunctional 2-component implant. The cells were incubated for 48hr. The statistical data was calculated according to [127].

4.4. Animal experiments

4.4.1. Surgery and implantation

Three animals (specific-pathogen-free rabbits; Charles River-WIGA, Sulzfeld; Germany) were operated under anesthesia as represented in scheme. (Figure 27) Briefly, the operation consisted in preparing carefully both rabbit femurs, avoiding dilapidation of muscles and tendons. Than, two artificial bone defects with 3 mm diameter were created in subcondrylic proximal and distal positions according to a predefined plan. (*see experimental section*) The two components (plastic-like filler matrix – PMSA – and PLASSM) were mixed before implantation in a ratio 1:100 resulting in the biofunctional 2-component implant. One artificial bone defects was filled with the bifunctional 2-component implant using a K-wire bender, whereas three others were used as controls containing PLASSM, PMSA, and a repetition of the any other component. The inner sutures were sewed with self-resolvent fibers and skin sutures ditto. After 9 weeks, the animals were sacrificed according to an approved procedure and the femurs removed and than fixated in a buffered solution containing 10% formalin until further analysis.

Results

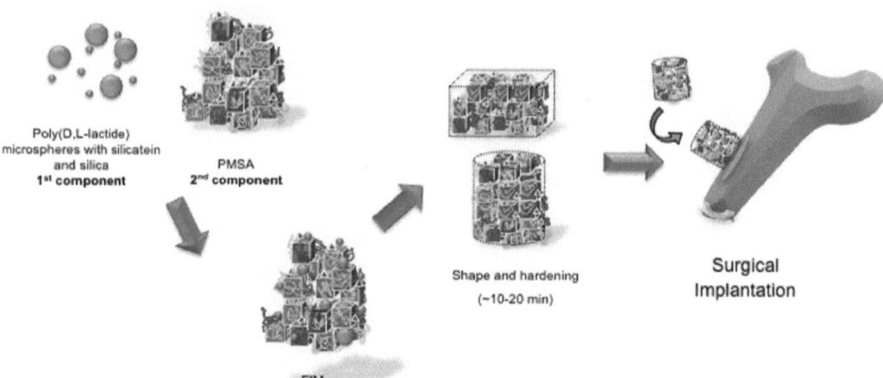

Figure 27. Schematic representation of implant preparation and surgical implantation into rabbit femur.

4.4.2. Computed tomography (CT) and micro-computed tomography (μ-CT) analysis of implant contrast within the bone

Two sets of control *ex vivo* experiments were performed. In the first set, an artificial bone defect with 3mm diameter (similar to the one performed during the surgical procedure) was created in rabbit femur, left open and further analyzed by Computed Tomography (CT). Figure 28 shows a set of cross-sections where the artificial bone defect can be easily visualized due to the difference in image contrast.

Results

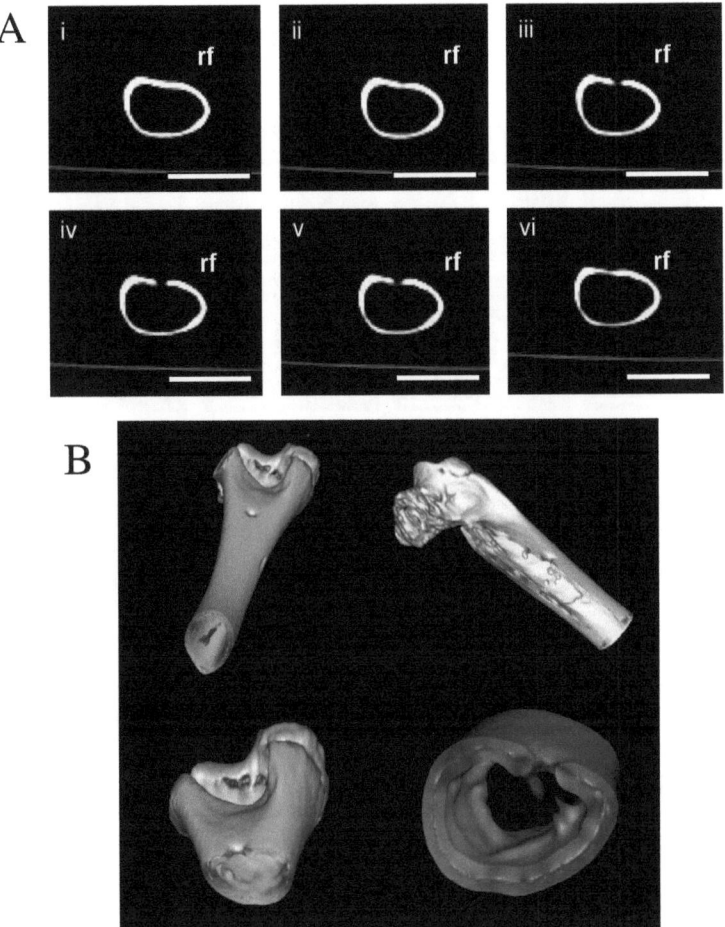

Figure 28. (**A**) Computed Tomography (CT) sequential images of cross sections of rabbit femur (*rf*) with an empty 3mm artificial bone defect (iii-v). Scale bar: 1 cm. (**B**) 3D reconstruction of rabbit femur.

In a second set of control experiments, an artificial bone defect (3mm) was created in a rabbit femur and filled with bifunctional 2-component implant. Analyzing successive cross-sections of the area that contains the implanted material it can be visualized that the material has a different image contrast when compared with natural bone contrast, (Figure 29 iii-v) making the bifunctional 2-component implant suitable for clinical control of bone regenerative evolution.

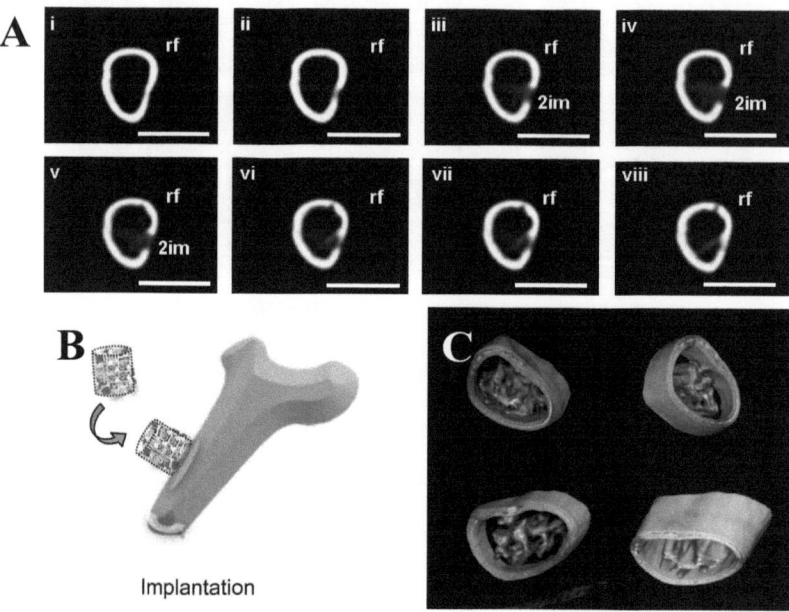

Figure 29. (**A**) Sequential Computed Tomography (CT) imaging of rabbit femur (*rf*) cross sections filled with containing bifunctional 2-compontent implant (*2im*) (iii-v). Implant and bone tissue show a different contrast (iii-v). Scale bar: 1 cm. (**B**) Implantation of bifunctional 2-compontent implant. (**C**) 3D reconstruction of rabbit femur.

Another tomographic analysis was carried out on this sample. For this purpose, rabbit femur containing the artificial bone defect filled with bifunctional 2-component implant was analyzed by micro-Computed Tomography (μ-CT). From Figure 30 there is clear a difference in materials (color difference), texture and morphology of bone tissue and implant.

Results

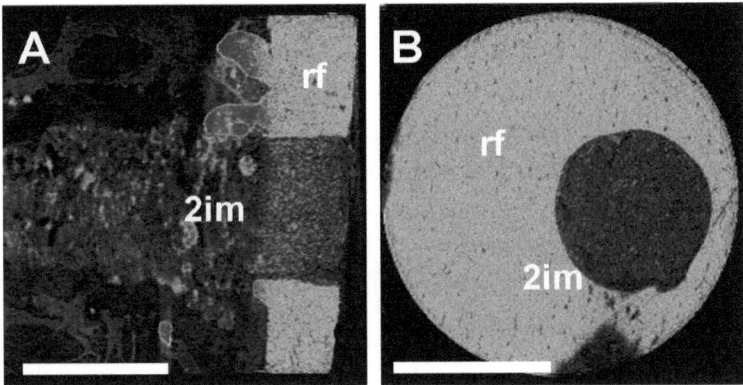

Figure 30. Micro-Computed Tomography (μ-CT) images of rabbit femur (*rf*) containing 2-compontent implant (*2im*) from different positions. (**A**) side view (**B**) upper view. Scale bar: 3mm.

4.4.3. Analysis of bone regenerative capacity after 9 weeks of implantation

Three rabbits were used for *in vivo* experiments and among the 6 femurs at least one artificial bone defects in each rabbit femur contained the bifunctional 2-component implant while the others were filled with the respective controls.

During the implantation period, all treated animals did not show any signs of abnormal behavior or physical deterioration. After 9 weeks, the animals were sacrificed, the 6 femurs removed and fixated in buffered solution containing 10% formalin and analyzed concerning surface scars and level of internal bone regenerations by digital imaging and Computed Tomography (CT), respectively. The results shown further, described only one animal experiment due to the similar results obtained for all the three different animals used.

4.4.3.1. External Morphology

The morphology of the rabbit femur surface, after 9 weeks of implantation, is shown in Figure 31. The arrows in the figure indicate the location where the artificial bone defect was created. Figure 31A shows the artificial bone defect performed in proximal position of the left rabbit's femur. This artificial bone defect was used as one of the controls and filled with PMSA, which is composed of silica amorphous microsized particles and polymers (PVP and starch). The image shows a scar that can be

Results

visualized as a small concavity/defect, clearly indicating that the regeneration was not complete. Another control experiment was performed using simply PLASSM to fill the artificial bone defect (3mm diameter) at the distal position of the left femur. (Figure 31B) Although the femur surface seemed to be less defective when compared to the bone defect filled with PMSA, a closer analysis shows the borders of the implant (white circle), indicating also incomplete bone regeneration.

Furthermore, two artificial bone defects (3 mm diamter) in rabbit right femur, both localized in distal and proximal positions, were filled with bifunctional 2-compontent implant. (Figure 31C and D) The combination of PMSA and PLASSM elicit the best results. In both cases, the scars at femur's surface, where the defects were previously created, are difficult to distinguish from the surrounding bone indicating completely surface recovery.

However, even if the surface analysis is here reported with good results, it would be important to determine whether implanted material is still present within the artificial defects or if it was reabsorbed and which is the degree of bone regeneration in the presence of these different materials (PMSA; PLASSM and 2-compontent implant). For this purpose Computed Tomography (CT) analysis was performed.

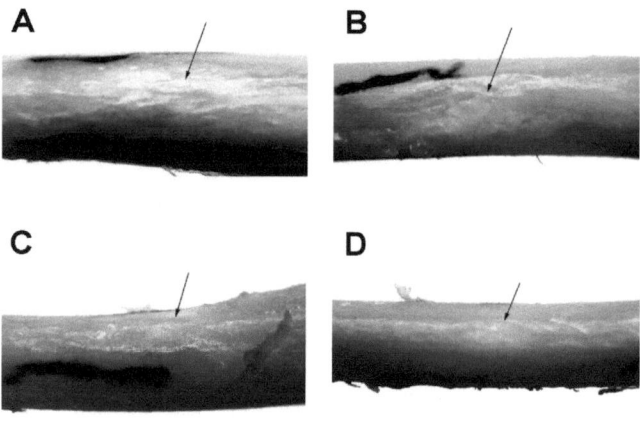

Figure 31. Photographic images of the rabbit femur's surface after 9 weeks post-implantation. The positions and corresponding implanted material are as follows: (**A**) left proximal – PMSA (**B**) left distal – PLASSM; (**C**) right proximal – bifunctional 2-compontent implant; (**D**) right distal – bifunctional 2-compontent implant. Arrows mark the places of surgical intervention.

4.4.3.2. Computed tomography (CT)

Computed tomography (CT) was performed in rabbit femurs (for the same samples described above) because is a *"non-destructive"* technique and therefore suitable in a first approach to analyze and evaluate the degree of bone regeneration. Unfortunately, it was not possible to follow implant behavior (resorption for example) and bone regeneration level *in vivo* during the complete time of implantation (9 weeks). Using the bifunctional 2-component implant, and its intrinsic characteristics under the CT (and X-rays), has previously shown it would have been possible to track the regeneration process without sacrificing the animal.

The set of CT images showed in Figure 32 represents cross-sections of rabbit femurs (left/right and/or distal/proximal) with artificial defects (3 mm diameter) that were implanted with different implant material. However, due to the difficulty in locating the scars under CT, especially in the right femur (in both distal and proximal positions), a needle containing a common CT contrast agent had to be positioned on top of the femurs exactly at the scars position (not shown). Moreover, the CT image quality was set to its highest resolution (1024x1024). Figure 32A shows the CT image of the left proximal position. No signal regarding the PMSA can be observed in the image. However, a small cavity and some bone deformation (Figure 32A, white arrow) were observed, in agreement with the morphological analysis (Figure 32A) reinforcing the idea of incomplete bone regeneration. No other pathological alterations of the normal bone structure are observed (e.g. hypercalcification). On the same way, when the PLASSM is introduced into the artificial defect an imperfect regeneration is also observed under the CT, corroborating the results obtained with the surface analysis. (Figure 32B) Due to the lack of contrast of PLASSM under CT it becomes difficult to evaluate the presence (or absence) of the material and histological analysis would be required to further evaluate the degree of regeneration and implant material resorption. In this case, hypercalcification of the bone or other bone pathologies are also absent.

The CT images of the right rabbit femur, both from proximal and distal positions where the artificial defects were created and filled with bifunctional 2-compontent implant (*2im*), show a clear lack of contrast signal indicating a complete absence of material within bone tissue after the implantation period indicating that the material has been resorbed by the organism. (Figure 32C and D) Again, no pathological alterations of the bone are observed. These CT images are also in agreement with previously images obtained by the digital images (Figure 32C and D) where surface deformation is completely absent, suggesting an increased level of bone regeneration. The 3D reconstruction of the rabbit bone shows complete bone regeneration.

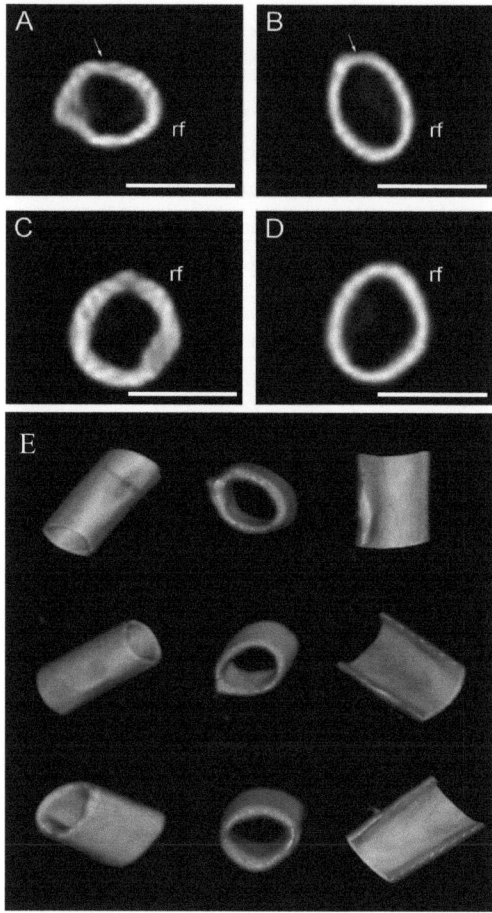

Figure 32. Computed tomography (CT) analysis of the rabbit femur (*rf*) implanted with different materials 9 weeks post-implantation. The positions and corresponding implanted material are as follows: (**A**) left proximal – PMSA (**B**) left distal – PLASSM; (**C**) right proximal – bifunctional 2-compontent implant; (**D**) right distal – bifunctional 2-compontent implant. White arrows mark the places of surgical intervention. Scale bar: 1 cm. (**E**) 3D reconstruction.

5. Discussion

The standard procedure for bone reconstruction has been, for many decades, the use of grafts from various donors and human body skeletal regions. However, these transplantation procedures are hampered by limited availability of donors, morbidity during bone harvesting process [137, 138] and the risk of disease transmission.[139] Despite these obstacles, bone grafts remain more effective (also called the *gold standard*) then when compared to artificial bone substitutes currently available. Bone grafts provide both osteoinductive and osteoconductive properties, where most artificial bone substitutes do not meet these requirements.[99] The low availability of donors and the increased demand of an elderly population, in combination with the risk of disease transmission, brings many researchers worldwide to explore new pathways for the development of new bone replacements, using a synthetic approach to fabricate materials (biomaterials) that aims to meet all the requirements, i.e., biomimicking the natural bone in all its features.[99]

Extraordinarily, the natural product biosilica, silica produced enzymatically under mild conditions (e.g. silicatein), comprises osteoinductive properties but not necessarily osteoconductive.[64, 65] Silicatein was isolated from sponge spicules, cloned, and prepared in a recombinant way so that its catalytic activity is preserved.[35, 131] Within the view that a deep understanding of biomineralization processes and the resulting natural products inspires the development of new biomaterials, a bifunctional 2-component implant biomaterial was generated, comprising encapsulated active silicatein (osteoinductive) and a silica-based solid matrix (osteoconductive) for application in the field of bone regeneration. Thus, silicatein was successfully encapsulated together with its substrate (sodium metasilicate, SM) into polymeric microspheres [poly(D,L-lactide)/polyvinylpyrrolidone microspheres (PLASSM)], using the classical methodology of w/o/w emulsion with solvent casting, in order to: (i) protect the protein that would undergo immediate proteolytic degradation immediately after entering body environment, (e.g., immune defense mechanism and proteolytic enzymes); and (ii) promote its controlled release upon implantation into the bone defect, creating a very peculiar microenvironment propitious to the formation of biosilica leading ultimately to cell recruitment, expansion, differentiation and bone regeneration. Furthermore, osteoconductivity was explored by designing a solid support that comprises amorphous silica particles, cross-linked with biodegradable (pore forming – macroporous structure) and biocompatible polymers (PMSA) that constitute a suitable and almost natural environment for the enzyme. Silicatein contains a specific site in its 3D structure (serine cluster) that targets specifically silica surfaces, maintaining its conformational integrity, essential for its catalytic activity in forming osteoinductive biosilica biopolymers.

Finally, the combination of these two components (PLASSM and PMSA) forms a material with adjustable, controllable, and hardening properties suitable for clinical applications. Preliminary *in vivo* experiments, performed in female athymic rabbit's femurs, revealed complete bone regeneration with complete resorption of the bifunctional 2-component implanted material after 9 weeks, contributing to a successful introduction of biosilica-based implants into the fields of bone substitution and regeneration.

5.1. Microencapsulation of silicatein and respective precursor (sodium metasilicate) into poly(D,L-lactide) biodegradable microspheres

Biodegradable polymers (both synthetic and natural derived) have been extensively investigated in tissue engineering, for example, to provide controlled release of therapeutic proteins, vaccine antigens, and small bioactive molecules, varying from days to months.[140]

Poly(D,L-lactide) (PLA) is by far the most used polymer in tissue engineering since its initial use in the early 70's has biodegradable suture fibres to nano- or microparticle-based delivery systems.[141-144] PLA is commercially available, FDA (United States Food and Drug Administration Agency) approved, and well known for its successful applications in the medical field. It finds application in tissue engineering scaffolds or drug-delivery systems, with a specially focus on bone regeneration (e.g., bone substitutes) due to its biocompatibility, processibility, biodegradability, and controlled cargo release.[145] However, PLA-based drug-delivery systems face two major limitations during protein encapsulation process: (i) possible deactivation of the enzyme during encapsulation (e.g., through exposition to organic solvents – PLA is hydrophobic) and (ii) formation of an acidic microenvironment in the vicinity of the polymer during drug release, due to polymer degradation, that leads to destabilization of acid-labile bio-macromolecules.[146, 147]

Encapsulation of small organic molecules or peptides such as paclitaxel [148], salicylic acid [149], bone morphogenic proteins (BMP) [146, 150, 151], and growth factors [146, 152-154] has been successfully achieved using PLA-based methodologies and it is well documented. However, enzyme encapsulation in PLA-based systems has remained a challenge, i.e., reduced activity immediately after the first step of encapsulation (i.e., contact with organic solvents) and a very low encapsulation yield.[155] In order to overcome this limitation, the synthesis of amphiphilic block co-polymers (PEG and PLA) has been described, only very recently, to successfully encapsulate an enzyme (catalase) that

Discussion

retained its full enzymatic activity after being processed using the classic approach of double emulsion.[156] Nevertheless, the synthesis of this type of polymers is not only laborious but also costly, making it difficult to find its application in the medical field when considering a upscale production.

In order to overcome the second major limitation (e.g. acidic microenvironment), several approaches have been used. For example, co-encapsulating poorly water-soluble slightly alkaline additives such as $Mg(OH)_2$, together with bovine serum albumin (BSA) or therapeutic proteins (e.g. recombinant human basic fibroblast growth factor [bFGF] or bone morphogenetic protein-2 [BMP-2]) have been demonstrated to remain stable and undamaged for more than 1 month.[146, 157] Another successful approach using a blend of slowly degrading poly(D,L-lactide) and water-soluble poly(ethylene glycol) (PEG) that reduced the production of acidic species derived from polymer degradation during protein release, consequently increasing protein diffusion by an accelerated polymer degradation (e.g., dissolution of PEG).[158]

In the present study, for the first time an enzyme (silicatein) has been encapsulated in poly(D,L-lactide) (PLA) by using a classical water/oil/water (w/o/w) double emulsion system and solvent casting.[159] In order to overcome the above described limitations and avoid protein denaturation upon organic solvent exposition, the protein was first pre-emulsified in a polymeric matrix - polyvinylpyrrolidone (PVP). To the best of our knowledge, the use of a pre-emulsifing step, i.e., using PVP polymer prior to protein encapsulation in PLA has never been described. The only report found where a similar approach is used describes protein encapsulation within PLGA microspheres using the biopolymer starch and poly(ethylene glycol) (PEG) as a protein micronization adjuvant in a classical w/o/w emulsion.[160]

Polyvinylpirrolidone (PVP) is an amphiphilic polymer derived from the monomer N-vinyl pyrrolidone. PVP is non-toxic, non-ionic, and widely used in pharmaceutical products. Several chemical modifications of PVP have also been described with multiple medical applications (e.g. Betadine – iodinated derivative). The pre-emulsion of silicatein with PVP results in electrostatic interactions (i.e. van der Waals forces and/or hydrogen bonds) between the protein and the PVP and in this way silicatein can be "trapped" within the polymeric matrix, avoiding direct contact with the organic solvent (methylene chloride) and consequent denaturation. It has been shown that polar carbonyl groups of PVP are responsible for interaction with other polar compounds through hydrogen bonding and this could be very likely the case that the presence of polar silicatein amino acids present at the surface of the protein interacts with PVP upon exposition.[161-165]

Upon this pre-emulsifying step, silicatein-PVP complex was added drop wise to a poly(D,L-

Discussion

lactide) solution (prepared in methylene chloride) in order to create polymeric microspheres. A brief sonication step was included, in order to create microspheres and carefull was taken to avoid protein denaturation. The solution was then poured into a stabilizer solution (PVP) and left at room temperature in order to evaporate the organic solvent (solvent casting). In our study, PVP was used as microsphere-stabilizer since it is (i) non-toxic; (ii) biocompatible; (iii) amphiphilic and (iv) polar. PVP can have a hydrophilic character, adsorbing exceptionally well to polar molecules and/or polymers, as for example, to PLA.[166] PVP association on the polymeric microspheres surface reduces significantly its hydrophobicity (PLA is highly hydrophobic) and enhances its biological applicability.[166, 167]

The choice of a stabilizer is of major importance in the field of tissue engineering scaffold design, since the stabilizer does not only regulate interaction between polymer and outer environment - and thus controls the drug release rate [168] - but it is also the first contact point with the cells limiting *a priori* its biomedical success. Several possible stabilizers, such as poly(vinyl alcohol) (PVA), polyethylene glycol (PEG), amphiphilic polymers (PVP), other polymers with surfactant properties (e.g. Poloxamers) and the typical surfactants (e.g., sodium dodecyl sulfate [SDS], cetyltrimethylammonium bromide bromide [CTAB)]) are commercially available and commonly used for this purpose. However, in particular SDS and CTAB do not find application in the medical field due to their high toxicity.[169] It is known that surfactants (SDS, CTAB, among others) interfere with cellular metabolism through their protein denaturating effects, ultimately leading to cell death.[169] Upon silicatein encapsulation, it was observed by means of immunostaining techniques that the enzyme (silicatein) is completely absent from the microsphere's surfaces and corroborating the idea that surface coatings of nonionic polymers such as poly(vinyl pyrrolidone) (PVP), poly(vinyl alcohol) (PVA), poly(vinyl methyl ether) (PVME), dextran, and methyl-cellulose reduce effectively surface adsorption of certain proteins (β-lactoglobulin and bovine serum albumin).[168]

After protein encapsulation, attempts to recover silicatein in order determine the incorporation of protein into the polymeric microspheres revealed to be unsuccessful. These attempts include (i) submission of PLASSM to preparative SDS-PAGE (inducing protein extraction by applying a direct electric field) [170] and (ii) dissolution of PLASSM in an organic solvent with subsequent extraction into an aqueous phase. Upon SDS-PAGE no protein could be detected, indicating that the presence of SDS and β-mercaptoethanol as well as heat treatment (95°C) were not sufficient to liberate the protein from the polymeric microspheres. Neither could dissolution of PLASSM in an organic solvent retrieve the enzyme, as determined by the application of Bradford methodology (Coomassie Blue stain) to the aqueous solution. This is not a complete unexpected result. Exposure of enzymes (carbonic anhydrase

Discussion

and horseradish peroxidase) encapsulated into PLGA-based microparticles to an organic/aqueous phase resulted in incomplete recovery of the protein due to its accumulation at the organic/aqueous phase interface. [171, 172] In our case, we can attribute the absence of silicatein in the aqueous solution to a similar behavior, i.e., water/organic solvent interface protein entrapment. To overcome these unsuccessful attempts, the presence of silicatein within the PLASSM was determined by immunodetection analysis and for this purpose, PLASSM were placed into a methylene chloride solution, briefly sonicated and spotted onto a membrane and treated with anti-silicatein polyclonal antibodies (PoAb-ASILIC).[9] The results show that the protein antibody recognition site was still intact as confirmed by a positive cross-reaction on the dot-blot.

Once the presence of silicatein within microspheres was proven, the encapsulation efficiency was further determined. Protein encapsulation efficiency is conventionally performed by the classical method based on the difference of protein recovery after encapsulation using Bradford methodolody (protein Coomassie blue stain). This approach has been extensively described for model proteins such as BSA [173] superoxide dismutase (SOD) and catalase [174], lysozyme [175] or horseradish peroxidase (HRP).[172] The presence of a pre-emulsifying step conditioned the use of this approach in our encapsulating methodology as no signal could be observed. Consequently, colorimetric densitometry of the detected spots on the dot-blot was performed, showing an encapsulation efficiency of $40\pm2\%$. In general, the efficiency of encapsulation of any protein into PLA-based structures (microspheres or surfaces) varies from 100% to 5 %, depending on the methodology of encapsulation as well as on the polymers and proteins used.

In a parallel approach, silicatein encapsulation was immunologically demonstrated by employing thin slices (50 μm) of PLASSM and applying PoAb-ASILIC. Microscopically analysis showed distribution of the protein within the PLASSM. This is the first report of such an approach. Additionally, the presence of silicatein within the microspheres was evaluated using fluorescein isothiocyanate (FITC)-labeled silicatein. Silicatein was labeled with a fluorophore (FITC) and the polymeric microspheres generated using the classical w/o/w with solvent casting. Afterwards, the microspheres were observed under a epifluorescent microscope and a clear green fluorescent signal is observed. This approach was already successfully employed using the model protein bovine serum albumin (FITC-BSA) encapsulated in PLA [176] and PLGA.[177]

Another goal in the development of biocompatible and biodegradable polymeric microspheres (PLASSM) containing silicatein, was the concurrent encapsulation of a non-toxic silicatein substrat. Sodium metasilicate (SM) is an inorganic monomer (SiO_4), water soluble with only a weak acidic pKa of 9.8, and poorly soluble in methylene chloride.[178] For this reason, sodium metasilicate (SM) turned out to be easy to encapsulate as confirmed by elemental analysis (EDX) of the loaded PLA-microspheres. So far, this is the first report on silica encapsulation within PLA-based microstructures.

5.2. Release of silicatein from polymeric microspheres (PLASSM)

The release rate of silicatein from PLASSM was conducted by immersing the polymeric microparticles either in simulated body fluid (SBF) or distilled water for a period of 15 days at a constant temperature (37°C). Simulated body fluid (SBF) was preferentially chosen, among other possible solutions (such as phosphate buffered solution [PBS]), due to the fact that SBF (i) mimics human serum mineral composition and (ii) for its ability to form an apatite layer in the presence of certain materials, the so called bioactivity.[128] A bioactive material in bone regeneration field is, by definition, a material that promotes *in vivo* apatite nucleation, with further growth (layering), leading to protein adsorption and consequently to cell adhesion, ingrowth and differentiation. In parallel, it creates a strong bond with the surrounding tissue culminating in bone regeneration. SBF is also known as the standard tool to test the bioactivity of implanting material and there seems to be a very close relationship between *in vitro* bioactivity of a material in the presence of SBF and its bioactivity *in vivo*.[179] Upon incubation for 15 days at 37°C with SBF, the formation of apatite on the surface of PLASSM was not observed on the surface of the polymeric material, suggesting that PLASSM is not bioactive and thus not masking the osteinductive role of silicatein in a further *in vivo* experiment. These results are in agreement with previous studies where it has been shown that PLA is not bioactive but PLA-based materials bioactivity can be achieved by addition of bioactive materials such hydroxyapatite [180, 181], TiO_2 [182, 183] or bioactive glass particles.[184, 185]

The release of silicatein under SBF conditions was carried out in parallel to the previous bioactivity studies, using an immuno-based assay (ELISA). The data shows that after 15 days only 15% of the total encapsulated silicatein has been released, suggesting that this release is a slow and continuous process. From these results, no initial release burst is observed. It has been shown that initial burst of protein release from PLA-based materials is directly co-related with protein adsorption-desorption processes at the surface of the polymeric microspheres.[186] The results obtained for silicatein release after SBF incubation are in agreement with aforementioned immuno-localization studies previously described, i.e., silicatein is located exclusively within the polymeric microspheres. Morphological inspection of PLASSM demonstrated that upon 15 days of incubation at 37°C in SBF, the polymeric microspheres change their morphology into bulky/fused polymeric material indicating that upon PLASSM dissolution, its cargo (protein) is released and the material can be resorped by the organism.

Discussion

PLA is a hydrophobic polymer with very slow degradation rate in aqueous solutions due to the methyl group of lactic acid that sterically protects the ester bonds of the polymer backbone from hydrolysis. The presence of PVP (amphiphilic polymer) at the surface of the PLASSM significantly reduces PLA hydrophobicity and, consequently, renders itssurface more hydrophilic and more susceptible to ionic attack.[168] The most common approach for studying the kinetics of drug release from PLA-based carriers, its co-polymers, and other linear polyesters involves the use of phosphate-based buffer solution (PBS, pH 7.2-7.4) at human body temperature (37°C) and is co-related with the different chemical susceptibilities (e.g. chemical attack) of polymer backbone ester bonds to hydrolysis.[187, 189] In this context, it has been proposed that the drug release mechanism of PLA co-polymer (e.g. PLGA) is based on three major events: (i) diffusion (active or passive), (ii) polymer degradation, and/or (iii) osmosis.[190] According to the obtained results from immuno-based assay (ELISA), silicatein release mechanism in SBF is due preferentially to polymer degradation mechanism (e.g. bulk erosion) with an eventual and minor contribution of osmosis-mediated efflux. Although it was not possible to observed under the SEM, PLASSM pores might be present and thus allow certain ions and water molecules to move into the polymeric structure, dissolving partially its internal matrix through PVP dissolution, and increasing slightly silicatein releasing rate. However, the contribution of the aforementioned event is not significant as shown by the control experiments, i.e., when PLASSM were incubated with distilled water only 7% of total encapsulated silicatein is released after 15 days (at 37°C). SEM imaging confirmed these results and showed that the integrity of the PLASSM is maintained without an increase of pore size indicating that PLASSM are stable in water for long periods of time finding its applicability in long term storage and keeping silicatein in a stable "dormant" state.

The activity of silicatein was only possible to determine after SBF exposition and release. The conservation of enzyme activity of encapsulated silicatein is of major concern. As described above, during the encapsulation process, the interaction between organic solvent (methylene chloride) and protein might induce severe changes in the protein conformation, leading to a loss of catalytic activity. After incubation of PLASSM in SBF for 15 days at 37°C and the supernatant was retrieved by centrifugation, the protein concentration measured showing the presence of 8μg as in agreement with ELISA results. Than, the activity of silicatein measured by incubating the protein (2 μg) with sodium metasilicate (200 μM) using the classical molybdate assay.[132] Although this methodology has some drawbacks (high detection limits) and is dependent from the degree of silica polymerization (only monomers and dimers can be detected)[for review see: 191], this assay continues to be commonly used

Discussion

to determine the degree of silica polymerization independent of the silica precursors employed and it has been applied also for determining silicatein activity in the presence of tetraorthosilicate (TEOS).[8, 34, 131, 192, 193] Interestingly, the results show that silicatein retains 75% of its initial activity upon release from PLASSM in SBF upon the full incubation period, indicating that the pre-emulsion step performed with PVP successfully protects the protein from conformational changes and significant activity loss and that the encapsulation procedure does not influence, in long term, the inherent catalytic activity of the enzyme.

Here, sodium metasilicate (SM) (200µM) was used as silicatein substrate for the first time. Additional experiments were carried out to confirm that SM can be used as silicatein substrate bearing in mind its future biomedical applications. Sodium metasilicate (SM) is the most likely candidate for several reasons: (i) low toxicity – is classified by the Food and Drug Administration (FDA) as ``Generally Recognized as Safe" and (ii) its abundance in the oceans derived essentially from biogenic origins, i.e., deteriorated diatoms and marine sponges skeletal elements Although is not within the scope of this thesis to address the fundamental question of the catalytic activity of silicatein towards SM, a brief discussion is given below.

The catalytic activity of silicatein towards SM was determined using FT-IR ATR time coursing measurements. According to these results, silicatein (2µg) is able to form biosilica polymers when incubated with SM (100 µM) under physiological conditions (pH 7.4 and room temperature). Surprisingly, it was possible to observe a transient intermediate tetracoordinated structure bonded to serine at silicatein's active site contradicting the proposed mechanism that describes the involvement and the formation of Si-pentacoordinated transient intermediated as found in the presence of polysaccharides.[8, 194] Taken together, silicatein has been demonstrated to be able to use SM as its "natural substrate" to form biosilica polymers finding its application in the medical field.

5.3. Component B: Production of plastic-like filler matrix containing silicic acid (PMSA)

Fundamental investigations of human cell biology commonly rely on 2D cell-culture systems that do not accurately recapitulate the structure, function, or physiology of living tissues. Systems for 3D cultures exist but do not replicate the spatial distributions of oxygen, metabolites, and signaling molecules found in tissues. Microfabrication can create architecturally complex scaffolds for 3D cell cultures that circumvent some of these limitations. Within this view, our choice for the design of a novel 3D scaffold was based on the fact that silica is an essential non-toxic dietary component for humans in a broad range of concentrations.[63] In higher animals, it has been proposed that silica

Discussion

seems to have both a structural as well as a metabolic role.[194] However, these assumptions still remain a challenge and many studies have been carried out in order to understand the exact influence of silica on bone cells (osteoblasts) and consequently on tissue growth development and finally on bone regeneration. It has been proposed that the structural role of silica displays the function of a biological cross-linker that contributes to architecture and resilience of connective tissue. [195] Basically, silica is a constitutive part of the extracellular matrix composed of glycosaminoglycans and polyuronides where it occurs firmly bounded to the polysaccharide matrix, possibly covalently bounded as an ester-like bond (e.g., silonate). From the cellular/metabolic point of view, scavenger receptors (MARCO) have been identified in macrophages that appear to be responsible for silica uptake and further cell up-signaling.[196] So far, no similar cellular studies at this level have been carried out on osteoblasts.

The silica based scaffold developed within this study, termed plastic-like filler matrix containing silicic acid (PMSA), is the first report on a complex inorganic-organic material as solid and moldable supportive matrix that consists of silica particles, a water insoluble polymer (starch), PVP, and hydrogen phosphate. The silica particles (average size distribution 10 µm) have been obtained by lowering the pH of a solution of water glass, supplemented with polymers (PVP and starch). This allows the formation of essential cross-linkages and a homogenous silica particle size distribution as observed by the control experiments. If water glass is precipitated simply by lowering the pH, a heterogeneous size and shape distribution would be achieved, suggesting that the combination of polymers in a certain ratio is responsible for the final size and shape of the silica particles. Starch facilitates the final implant material to be cohesive and partial insoluble in aqueous solutions. PVP, in combination with starch, allows the matrix to get harder at a desired rate and to partially dissolve under aqueous conditions, consequently forming pores as result of the unordered packing of silica particles.[210] Hydrogen phosphate [$H_2PO_4^{2-}$] contributes to the formation of hydroxyapatite during cell metabolism and guarantees pH stability (at around 7.0) for more than 2 weeks, which is essential since silica monomers leaching of the silica particles continuously increases the pH. The final matrix is moldable and thus suitable for filling irregular osseous defects, independent of their size or location.

Despite the essential role of silica in bone formation, the use of silica-based biomaterials for bone regeneration is not very common, and mostly restricted to the application of bioglasses and its chemical variations.[120-123] Independent of its composition, bioglass concept displays an amazing bioactivity, biocompatibility, and osteoinductivity with formation of an initial, chemically driven apatite surface layer both *in vitro* and *in vivo* that promotes an excellent bone ingrowth.[122, 197] Only very recently, another type of silica-based biomaterials has become an emerging trend. Some silica mesoporous materials (e.g. SBA-15 and MCM-48) can soon find an application in the field of tissue engineering

Discussion

since they exhibit strong bioactivity and simultaneously can be used as drug carriers with a well defined pore size and controlled drug release kinetics. [198, 199] Contrary to bioglasses, no *in vivo* studies have been conducted so far. Additional punctual studies have been published. For example, Coradin *et al.* created hybrid materials that display a certain similarity with bone at organizational level by co-polymerization of silica precursors and collagen monomers.[200, 201] However, this approach did not meet further success due to the inability of collagen to precipitate silica monomers under physiological conditions, it is a non-porous material and its biocompatibility was never tested.

An approach that has met more success and included *in vivo* studies was the one-pot synthesis of silica-substituted hydroxyapatite (Si-HA) (0.8% Si substitution).[202, 203] Although this material seems to enhance bone development *in vivo* when compared to hydroxyapatite-based implants several concerns were raised due to the fact that the authors did not show the direct influence of silica on cell growth and its release from Si-HA structure.[204- 207] Furthermore, another punctual successful experiment carried out using silica-based materials and *in vivo* experiments was by coating bioglass (Bioverit ® II) with nanoporous silica layer with further implantation into mouse ear model. The results showed an extensive ear cartilage recovery.[208] More recently, a silica gel matrix doped with hydroxapatite nanocrystals is now commercially available under the name of Nanobone®. The authors claim that the silica based materials and the HA display an incredible regenerative capacity and body resorption after 5 weeks of implantation. [209] Further studies have shown that the material resorption is caused by osteoclast activity indicating that this material is not only biocompatible and biodegradable but it capable of inducing a response from the organism in recruiting leaving behind the idea of inert implantable biomaterials. [210]

Despite the lack of one or another missing characterization from these new biomaterials, all the above described silica-based materials seem to be an excellent alternative to currently used biomaterials in bone regenerative medicine. Our bifuncional 2-component implant is in line with this material with an additional fact that carry osteoinductive materials derived from biomineralization processes.

One of the physical properties required of moldable matrices is the hardening time (working time), which greatly decides about the possible biomedical applicability of new biomaterials. In this study, the ratio of polymer blend (PVP and starch) was determined on basis of a surgical intervention, where 15-30 min is the required time between generating an artificial femur defect and subsequent implantation of the material. However, the ratio of these polymers can be altered accordingly giving to this material an incredible flexibility on setting the working time. One advantage of the proposed process is that it does not involve chemical reactions (e.g. photopolymerization, radical initiators) for polymerization/hardening to occur as described for other approaches [211, 212] air-drying and promotion of the cross-linkages between the silica amorphous microparticles is sufficient. In addition, due to its inherent properties, PMSA can be easily sterilized, inserted into a sterile syringe or implanted directly into the bone defect, consequently avoiding air-exposure and microbial/viral contamination.

This 4-component scaffold is easy to develop from the experimental point of view (room temperature, short time of preparation *ca.* 20 min), offering several advantages such biocompatibility, adequate/adjustable time of hardening, easy to sterilized and the possibility to be injectable minimizing possible contamination risks. Additionally, PMSA works as solid inorganic-organic support (for PLASSM for example or other components).

5.4. Bifunctional 2-component implant

Tissue engineering as been described, in its many different forms, as an emerging area directed towards the design of new materials than can help an organism to improve its ability of regeneration by recovering both structure and function of a lost or failed organ/tissue.[213] The most commonly used and safe approach was termed *neomorphogenesis* in the late 80's.[214] It comprises cell harvesting directly from the organ of the organism, cell culture, and expansion in bioreactors (depending on type of cells), co-incubation of cells with biocompatible and/or biodegradable scaffolds for cell attachment and proliferation, with eventual development into a functional tissue, followed by implantation of the scaffold-cell material into the host.[215] This approach was successfully used in regenerating different organs/tissues and has been refined during the last decades with the development of new polymeric matrices and new methodologies, new cell culture systems, or by encapsulation of cells in order to avoid undesired immunological reactions, where artificial pancreas and artificial liver represent the most recently examples.[216] However, optimal tissue engineering requires more than an inert scaffold to serve merely as a substrate for cell attachment and growth. In all cases, a scaffold that can interact and influence cellular behavior is of crucial importance. Most of the polymeric matrices have shown to be well tolerated by cells but signal molecules in the form of adhesion molecules, growth and differentiation factors should be incorporated into these scaffolds in a spatially defined manner to orchestrate the growth of new tissue.[215, 216] Additionally, in the case of hard implants (polymeric or metallic) it should provide mechanical support against compressive and tensile forces, maintaining the shape and integrity of the scaffold in the body's environment.

Another approach in tissue engineering that has been gaining great interest and attention among the scientific community is the increased understanding of general biomineralization processes. These have initiated new and interesting developments in biomimetic synthesis with generation and

Discussion

reproduction of biomimetic materials fabricated according to biological principles, for example, by mimicking structural features found in complex skeletal structures that occur widely in Nature.[217] Previous and current approaches that integrate natural products for biomedical applications are based on (i) marine derived biopolymers (e.g., alginates, chitosan) or (ii) biomineralization products (e.g., sea urchin spines, corals skeletons, nacre, spongin/collagen from marine sponges).[217] As far as to our knowledge, among the few silica-based materials only bioglasses, silica gel matrix doped with hydroxyapatite crystals (NanoBone®) and silica-substituted hydroxyapatite (Si-HA) (but not silica mesoporous materials) were successfully used *in vivo* but none introduces the concept of silica biomineralizating organisms.

The bifunctional 2-component implant developed in the context of this thesis is situated in between both approaches, comprising a moldable, hardening silica-based implant (inorganic) that acts as macroporous scaffolds (solid support) and a naturally occurring protein (silicatein) that is responsible for the synthesis of biosilica with osteoinductive properties.[64, 65]

The assessment of bifunctional 2-component implant bioactivity *in vitro* was performed in simulated body fluid (SBF) Upon incubation of the bifunctional 2-component with SBF for 15 days at body temperature (37°C) its morphology was inspected by SEM imaging. The images show a highly porous morphology that resembles that of a natural bone [218] with pore sizes varying from 500 nm up to several micrometers. These results indicate not only an interaction of SBF with silica-based scaffold (PMSA), inducing partial dissolution of the scaffold polymers (PVP and starch) and consequently creating pores, but also demonstrate that the initial architecture of the bifunctional 2-component implant (small pores between silica particles) is sufficient to allow the fluid to pass through. In a longer exposure to SBF, pores with larger size would be expected to be have been formed as a consequence of further matrix (PMSA) dissolution (both silica and cross-linking polymers), creating ideal conditions for cell invasion and proliferation. Pore formation within a scaffold is an important parameter for the design of implantable biomaterials for bone regenerative therapies. The size of the pores must be large enough to encourage cell migration and cell proliferation as it allows nutrients to diffuse, ultimately leading to tissue tridimensional development/growth (e.g., bone growth, vascularization, etc.). However, the concept of *optimal pore size* does not exist since bone has very different structures depending on function and localization. It stands to reason that the same pore size may not be ideal for all bone regeneration sites.[218-221]

The silica particles comprised into PMSA display slow dissolution rate (silica leaching) and do not induce the formation of apatite in the presence of SBF (e.g. bioinactive) Although, EDX was not performed, a closer SEM inspection showed the complete absence of the typical needle-like particles,

Discussion

indicative of initial stages of apatite formation. For example, the behavior of different macroporous silica materials under SBF elicits different reactions with each process displaying its own kinetics. SBA-15 develops the apatite layer after 30 days (in SBF) while 60 days are required in the case of MCM-48. Nevertheless, after 60 days of immersion the apatite layer did not appear in MCM-41.[222] It has been proposed that the presence (and quantity) of silanol groups (Si-OH) at the surface of the material is crucial for the bioactivity of silica-based materials, since they can act as nucleation sites for the formation of the apatite layer.[198] The lack of bioactivity of PMSA upon exposure to SBF might be due to the small amount of silanol groups present at the surface of the amorphous particles.

Our previous studies showed that silicatein is released from the polymeric microspheres (PLASSM) after SBF treatment. The possible location of released silicatein within the bifunctional 2-component implant (after SBF treatment) was evaluated through both immunochemistry as well as spectroscopic techniques (FT-IR ATR). Despite the fact that mature silicatein has an isoelectric point (IP) of 5.5 [9] and under normal physiological conditions (pH 7.2) displays a slightly negative overall net charge, becoming difficult to interact with the unshielded negatively charged silica particles (PMSA) except if via very specific protein-silica surface interactions. Attempts to functionalize directly silica nanospheres with urease by adsorption was not feasible, showing that not all enzymes have affinity for silica surfaces.[223] The silicatein sequence comprises a serine (Ser) cluster [10] that is responsible for anchoring the protein to silica surfaces. Recently studies showed that chemical modification of serine cluster with phenylmethylsulfonyl fluoride prevents adsorption to silica nanoparticles confirming the essentiality of this cluster for protein–silica interaction.[224]

The immunochemical analysis clearly indicate the presence of silicatein, which is widespread within the macroporous structure of the bifunctional 2-component implant. However, it was the FT-IR ATR analysis that brought additional and more conclusive results. The typical band for proteins in FT-IR spectrum contains peaks derived from amide bonds vibrations. The main band (amide I band) is centered at ~1600-1700 cm^{-1} and can be attributed to amide bond (C=O stretching vibrations). This band is sensitive to changes in secondary structure and has therefore been widely used for protein conformational studies.[225] FT-IR ATR analysis of bifunctional 2-component implant before SBF incubation shows a small band located at 1650 cm^{-1}, attributed to OH bending vibration modes that are commonly found in the same region of the amide I band. These hydroxyl groups might be derived from silanol groups (Si-OH) of silica particles (PMSA), and/or from the glycosyl groups of starch. The band located at 1750 cm^{-1} is attributed to stretch vibration modes of ketones, localized in a cyclic 5-membered ring. In this case, only the chemical structure of polyvinylpyrrolidone (PVP) matches the spectroscopic data. However, significant spectroscopic differences can be found after incubation of the

Discussion

bifunctional 2-component implant with SBF. Accordingly, a shift of amide I band from 1640 cm^{-1} (silicatein free state) to 1670 cm^{-1} suggests a change in the environment of the protein (protein backbone conformation) when compared with "free" silicatein. This small wavelenght shift observed on the FT-IR ATR spectrum suggests that silicatein can be classified as "hard" protein. This type of protein does not undergo significant conformational changes when adsorbed onto surfaces, in contrast to the so-called "soft" proteins (e.g. BSA).[226] Moreover, FT-IR ATR data indicate that silicatein retains its conformation (when compared with "free silicatein") upon release from the polymeric spheres and interaction with the silica surfaces.

The formation of biosilica through silicatein immobilized on the bifunctional 2-component implant was attempted. However, this task has shown to be extremely difficult to carry out as many factors are involved. It would have been interesting to distinguish between polyamorphs of precipitated silica particles and freshly formed biosilica. These techniques are, at the present time, not very well developed and involve complex and ambiguous analysis and thus no further analyses were carried out.

Additionally to protein adsorption analysis performed by FT-IR ATR, one interesting feature is present in spectrum after SBF incubation: two additional bands, located at 1510 and 1590 cm^{-1}. These bands can be assigned to symmetric and asymmetric stretching vibrations of deprotonated carboxylic acid groups originated from the degradation/hydrolysis of PLA-based microspheres by interaction of ions with the polyester backbone as described above confirming the results obtained from the protein release studies. It has been described that one of the limitations in using polyesters as scaffolds for tissue engineering is that their degradation originate an acidic microenvironment destabilizing acid-labile bio-macromolecules.[146] However, the addition of polymers such as PEG or slight alkaline compounds (e.g. Mg(OH)$_2$) circumvents this undesirable polymeric degradation side-effect. In case of the bifunctional 2-component implant the presence of silica particles with a certain alkaline character, PVP and an alkaline salt (Na$_2$HPO$_4$) play an important role on deleting the microenvironment acidity caused by PLA degradation.

5.4.1. Cytoxicity studies

Another important property of any implantable material is its biocompatibility, i.e., its interaction with living cells. Although not much work has been done so far using silica-based materials for medical applications (except bioglass, Si-HA and NanoBone®), it has been shown that amorphous silica is an essential nutrient for humans, especially to bone development, contrary to crystalline silica (e.g. quartz) that provokes diseases such as *silicosis* (lung disease due to the accumulation of crystalline silica particles.[61, 62, 121] Within this view, XRD analysis of the PMSA showed an amorphous structure

Discussion

indicating that the bulk material of the bifunctional 2-component implant can be safely used in biomedical application.

For this reason it not surprising to find that none of the silica-based materials in use for bone regenerative medicine do not show any cytotoxicity (and toxicity).[107, 120-123, 202, 203, 209] Interestingly was the fact that that co-incubation human osteosarcoma cell line MG-63 with orthosilicate (SiO_4) (up to 50µM) does not only displays no cytotoxicity but it also promotes expression of osteoblast differentiation markers (e.g. osteocalcin), alkaline phosphatase and collagen type I up to 2-fold.[227, 228] In a similar way, biosilica also induces osteoblast differentiation by strong gene up-regulation of sialoprotein, osteocalcin, and osteoponctin in SaOS-2 cells (human osteosarcoma) but up to 4-fold. Moreover, studies conducted on silicatein and biosilica biocompatibility have shown that the enzyme and its product is non-toxic to cells and organisms.[229]

The biocompatibility of the bifunctional 2-component implant was assessed using HEK293 and Chinese hamster ovary cells (7WD10). These results show that that this composite material is non-toxic as well as non-proliferative and does not display differentiation property (osteoinductive) for both cell lines. Interesting was the fact that when SaOS-2 and PDL-fibroblasts cell lines were co-incubated with bifunctional 2-component implant did not only show no cytotoxicity but it also promotes cell proliferation (ingrowth) increased gene activation and up-regulation (e.g. osteocalcin). However, when the bifunctional 2-component implant without PLASSM was used as control, the cells retain their viability and no gene expression occurred. The Si-bioactivity specificity induction in certain cells can be attributed to the nutrient requirement (in this case Si) of certain cells (osteoblasts and fibroblasts) to perform their metabolic functions.

Taken together, the 2-component implant and all its components (PVP, PLA, silicatein, starch) does not show toxicity towards different cell lines (SaOS-2, PDL-fibroblasts, HEK293, 7WD10) and can be classified as biocompatible, biodegradable, and bioactive specific composite material, with significant potential contribution to bone mineralization and regeneration.

5.5. Bifunctional 2-component implant: *ex vivo* and *in vivo* studies

5.5.1. *Ex vivo* studies

Several techniques were used to evaluate the physical properties of the bifuctional 2-component implant, such as micro-computed tomography (µ-CT), X-ray's and Computed Tomography (CT). Surprisingly, the bifuctional 2-component implant was detected under X-ray and CT analysis. *Ex-vivo* implants were conducted by filling an artificial defect (3 mm), created in a female rabbit femur, with a pre-hardened bifuctional 2-component implant. The micro-Computed Tomography (µ-CT) images show a difference in contrast and morphology when compared with the natural bone indicating that µ-CT is a suitable technique for evaluation of the level of bone regeneration. However, this technique is not so widely used and requires costly machinery.

On the other hand, CT results showed different image contrast between the cortical bone and the implanted material suggesting that a continuous clinical analysis (bone regeneration level) after femur implantation can be easily performed in any near hospital avoiding additional surgical interventions and, if necessary, adjust the treatment accordingly.

5.5.2. *In vivo* preliminary studies

Bone tissue is unique in that it retains a high regenerative capacity. However, due to its complexity in structure and composition, the regeneration of bone defects, regardless their origin (e.g. congenital, tumor), through implants remains difficult. Biocompatible, biodegradable, osteoinductive, and moldable implant materials are favorable to bone cement fillers that simply seal the defect. To evaluate the bifunctional 2-component implant in *in vivo,* artificial defects (3 mm diameter) were created in distal and proximal position of rabbit femurs. Three female athymic rabbits were carefully prepared under surgery ethical procedures and an artificial bone defects created (3 mm diameter). The bifunctional 2-component was implanted as well as the respective controls. After implantation procedure was carried out, the artificial bone defects were sutured and the animal kept under normal conditions for 9 weeks. None of the treated animals showed any signs of abnormal behavior or physical deterioration during the implantation period suggesting that the material is non-toxic, does not induce any pathological alterations and thus is well tolerated by the organism. After 9 weeks, the animals were sacrificed, according to the ethical procedure, and the femurs analyzed.

The morphological analysis of surface of the femur cicatrisation and CT analysis show that the untreated defect (control) displays an incomplete regeneration with formation of a concavity at the surface of the femur, confirming the auto-regenerative capacity of bone. However, this healing process is still incomplete after 9 weeks. At this stage, hypercalcification or other severe malformations are not observed. In the second control experiments, using the bifunctional 2-component implant that had not been supplemented with PLASSM, also an incomplete regeneration is observed. The same results can be found for the control experiment carried out using only PLASSM as defect filler. On the other hand, analysis of the femur implanted with the complete bifunctional 2-component material showed that the surface scar is minimal and less extensive compared to the controls and that the bone is complete regenerated.

Discussion

Additionally, CT analysis demonstrated the absence of PMSA (control) and bifunctional 2-component implant after 9 weeks, indicating that the silica-based material is completely resorbed. These results are in agreement with the only other silica-based bone implant material available (e.g. Nanobone®). The authors describe that the silica gel matrix, doped with nanocrystalline hydroxyapatite (n-HA) is non-toxic for osteoblasts, osteoclasts and fibroblasts, stimulates collagen production and bone growth, and is replaced *in vivo* by an organic matrix within 5 weeks (Götting minipigs). Moreover, the same authors recently attributed the silica degradation is promoted by osteoclasts during bone remodeling processes.[209,210]

As previously observed, if on one side PMAS is neither osteoinductive nor bioactive, does not induce cell proliferation it can be classified as an inert solid polymeric-inorganic supportive guiding matrix. On the other side, PLASSM is also neither cytotoxic nor the PLA shell is bioactive but it contains silicatein that can form osteoinductive biosilica and but does not have an osteoconductive property. These aforementioned results indicate that PLASSM or PMSA *per se* are not sufficient to induce complete bone development and ingrowth and that complete bone regeneration is due to a synergetic effect of both PLASSM (and the presence of silicatein) and PMSA, i.e., bifunctional 2-component implant.

Finally, a schematic representation of the *modus operandi* of the bifunctional 2-component implant *in vivo* is proposed. (Figure 33) In the first step, the implant is prepared and introduced into the defect. After some time exposed to body fluids, two major events occur. The first the slow degradation of the matrix that leads to the formation of open pores and the second, the degradation of polymeric microspheres with consequent release of silicatein. Since the matrix is build up from silica, the release silicatein will attach to its surface via serine clusters promoting the formation of a biosilica layer. In turn, this newly formed layer will attract osteosblast that migrate through the pores and settle on this new layer. From this point, the normal bone regeneration process takes place. During this process the implanted material start to get replaced by newly formed bone and finally the bone is fully regenerated.

Discussion

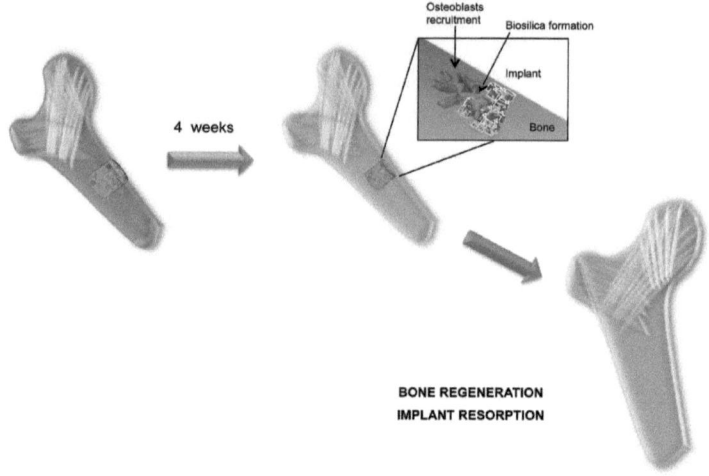

Figure 33. Schematic represention of *modus operandi* of the bifunctional 2-component implant *in vivo*.

6. Conclusion

For biomedical application of a novel functional implant materials (bifunctional 2-component implant) that aim to exploit the advantages of biosilica biopolymer, two major technological problems had to be circumvented: (i) the encapsulation of the active enzyme (osteoinductive properties) within biodegradable, biocompatible polymeric (PLA) microspheres in order to protect the enzyme from body environment (e.g. immune system, proteolyic enzymes, etc) (PLASSM) and (ii) the development of a biodegradable, biocompatible, silica-based matrix with adjustable hardening time (working time) with osteoconductive properties.

The first task has been successfully solved by encapsulating both silicatein ($40\pm2\%$ encapsulation efficiency) and its substrate (sodium metasilicate) into PLA-microspheres in a classical w/o/w double emulsion methodology with solvent casting and using PVP both as pre-emulsifying and stabilizer polymer. The PLASSM did not show to be bioactive under biomimetic conditions, no cytotoxicity to any of the components and displayed a controlled and slow release of silicatein with activity retention (75%) upon release. In the second task, a multifunctional matrix was developed to entrap PLASSM, consisting of a polymer blend of PVP and starch embedded into a silica-based material. These components did not show any bioactivity or cytotoxicity when co-incubated under biomimetic conditions indicating its suitability for further biomedical applications.

Subsequently, the bifunctional 2-component implant was successfully employed to treat artificial defects in athymic rabbit femurs, resulting in both bone complete regeneration and resorption of the implanted material after nine weeks. None of the treated animals revealed pathological lesions or symptoms and neither silicatein nor bifunctional 2-component implant demonstrated adverse effects in animal toxicity assays.

In conclusion, bifunctional 2-component implant highly qualifies for application as a potential silica-based bone replacement/substitution material inspired in biomineralization processes for regenerative medicine since it is (i) biodegradable, (ii) biocompatible, (iii) adjustable working time without the use of chemical reactions, (iv) solid silica matrix that has osteoconductive properties and (v) contains silicatein and its substrate, both of which facilitate the synthesis of biosilica with osteoinductive activity.

7. Bibliography

[1] J.T. Baker, V. Murphy, *CRC Handbook of Marine Science*, CRC Press, BocaRaton, USA, 1981

[2] W.E.G. Müller, R.K. Zahn, K. Bittlingmeier, D. Falke, *Ann. New York Acad. Sci.*, 284, 34-48, 1977

[3] H.A. Lowenstam, S. Weiner, *On Biomineralization*, Oxford University Press, Oxford, 1989

[4] S. Weiner, P.M. Dove, *Rev. Min. & Geochem.*, 54, 1-29, 2003

[5] X. H. Wang, W.E.G. Müller, *Frontiers of Materials Science in China (FMSC); in press*, 2009

[6] B.E. Volcani, In: T.L. Simpson, B.E. Volcani (eds), *Silicon and siliceous structures in biological systems*, Springer, New York, USA, 157-200, 1981

[7] W.E.G. Müller, X.H. Wang, S.I. Belikov, W. Tremel, U. Schloßmacher, A. Natoli, D. Brandt, A. Boreiko, M.N. Tahir, I.M. Müller, H.C. Schröder In: Bäuerlein E (ed) Handbook of Biomineralization Vol.1. *The Biology of Biominerals Structure Formation*. Wiley-VCH, Weinheim, Germany, 59-82, 2007

[8] J.N. Cha, K. Shimizu, Y. Zhou, S.C. Christianssen, B.F. Chmelka, G.D. Stucky, D.E. Morse, *Proc. Natl. Acad. Sci. USA*, 96,361-365, 1999

[9] W.E.G. Müller, M. Rothenberger, A. Boreiko, W. Tremel, A. Reiber, H.C. Schröder, *Cell Tissue Res.*, 321, 285-297, 2005

[10] W.E.G. Müller, K. Jochum, B. Stoll, X.H. Wang, *Chem. Mater.*, 20, 4703-4711, 2008

[11] X.H. Wang, A. Boreiko, U. Schloßmacher, D. Brandt, H.C. Schröder, J. Li, J.A. Kaandorp, H. Götz, H. Duschner, W.E.G. Müller, *J. Struct. Biol.*, 164, 270-280, 2008

[12] N. Kröger, R. Deutzmann and M. Sumper, *Science*, 286, 1129-1132, 1999

[13] G. Mayer, *Science*, 310, 1144-1147, 2005

Bibliography

[14] V. Donati, *Auszug seiner Natur-Geschichte des Adriatischen Meeres*. Francken, Halle, Germany, 1753

[15] P.S. Pallas, *Charakteristik der Thierpflanzen*. Raspiche Buchhandlung, Nürnberg, 1787

[16] R.E. Grant, *Lancet*, 1,153-159, 1833

[17] O. Schmidt, Grundzüge einer Spongien-Fauna des Atlantischen Gebietes.Gustav Fischer, Leipzig, 1870

[18] L.H. Hyman In: Hyman H (ed) *Invertebrates: Protozoa Through Ctenophora*. McGraw-Hill Book Co. Inc., New York, USA, 284-364, 1940

[19] B.A. Afzelium, *Nature*, 191, 4453-4456, 1961

[20] L. Salvini-Plawen, *Z. ZoolSyst. Evolutionsforsch.*, 16, 40-88, 1978

[21] W.E.G. Müller, *Naturwiss.*, 82, 321-329, 1995

[22] W.E.G. Müller, *Comp. Biochem. Physiol. (A)*, 129, 433-460, 2001

[23] G. Walker, *Snowball Earth: The story of the great global catastrophe that spawned life as we know it*. Crown Publishers, New York, USA, 2003

[24] S. Xiao, X. Yuan, A.H. Knoll, *Proc. Natl. Acad. Sci. USA*, 97, 13684-13689, 2000

[25] W.E.G. Müller, J. Li, H.C. Schröder, L. Qiao, X.H. Wang, *Biogeosci.*, 4, 219-232, 2007

[26] A.H. Knoll, S.B. Carroll, *Science*, 284, 2129-2137, 1999

[27] D. Nicol, *J. Paleontol.*, 40, 1397-1399, 1966

[28] X.H. Wang, H.C. Schröder,W.E.G. Müller, *Int. Rev. Cell. Mol. Biol.*, 273, 69-115, 2009

[29] C. Gesner, Historiae Animalium. Vol. 20. C Forer, Zürich, 1558

[30] W.E.G. Müller, X. Wang, F-Z. Cui, K. P. Jochum, W. Tremel, J. Bill, H. C. Schröder, F. Natalio, U. Schloßmacher and M. Wiens, *Appl. Microbio. Biotech*, 83, 397-413, 2009

[31] F. Sandford, *Microsc. Res. Tech.*, 62:336-355, 2003

[32] J.C. Weaver, L.I. Pietrasanta, N. Hedin, B.F. Chmelka, P.K. Hansma, D.E. Morse, *J. Struct. Biol.*, 144, 271-281, 2003

[33] A. Woesz, J.C. Weaver, M. Kazanci, Y. Dauphin, J. Aizenberg, D.E. Morse, P. Fratzl, *J. Mater. Res.*, 21, 2068-2078, 2006

[34] W.E.G. Müller, X.H. Wang, K. Kropf, H. Ushijima, W. Geurtsen, C. Eckert, M.N. Tahir, W. Tremel, A. Boreiko, U. Schloßmacher, J. Li, H.C. Schröder, *J. Struct. Biol.*, 161, 188–203. 2008

[35] W.E.G. Müller, U. Schloßmacher, X.H. Wang, A. Boreiko, D. Brandt, S.E. Wolf, W. Tremel, H.C. Schröder, *FEBS J.*, 275, 362-370, 2008

[36] H.C. Schröder, A. Krasko, G. Le Pennec, T. Adell, H. Hassanein, I.M. Müller, W.E.G. Müller, *Progr. Molec. Subcell. Biol.*, 33, 249-268, 2003

[37] W.E.G. Müller, X.H. Wang, K. Kropf, A. Boreiko, U. Schloßmacher, D. Brandt, H.C. Schröder, M. Wiens, *Cell Tissue Res.*, 333, 339-351, 2008

[38] H.C. Schröder, A. Boreiko, M. Korzhev, M.N. Tahir, W. Tremel, C. Eckert, H. Ushijima, I.M. Müller, W.E.G Müller, *J. Biol. Chem.*, 281, 12001-12009, 2006

[39] M.M. Murr, D.E. Morse, *Proc. Natl. Acad. Sci. USA*, 102, 11657-11662, 2005

[40] W.E.G. Müller, A. Boreiko, U. Schloßmacher, X.H. Wang, M.N. Tahir, W. Tremel, D. Brandt, J.A. Kaandorp, H.C. Schröder, *Biomaterials*, 28, 4501-4511, 2007

[41] M.R. Custódio, I. Prokic, R. Steffen, C. Koziol, R. Borojevic, F. Brümmer, M. Nickel, W.E.G. Müller, *Mech. Ageing Dev.*, 105, 45-59, 1998

[42] C. Eckert, H.C. Schröder, D. Brandt, S. Perovic-Ottstadt, W.E.G. Müller, *J. Histochem. Cytochem.*, 54, 1031-1040, 2006

Bibliography

[43] H.C. Schröder, S. Perovic-Ottstadt, M. Rothenberger, M. Wiens, H. Schwertner, R. Batel, M. Korzhev, I.M. Müller, W.E.G. Müller, *Biochem. J.*, 381, 665-673, 2004

[44] E. Mugnaioli, F. Natalio, U. Schloßmacher, X.H. Wang, W.E.G. Müller, U. Kolb,. *ChemBioChem*, 10, 683-689, 2009

[45] G. Imsiecke, W.E.G. Müller, *Cell. Mol. Biol.*, 41, 827-832, 1995

[46] M. Maldonado, C. Carmona, M.J. Uriz & A. Cruzado, *Nature*, 401, 785-788, 1999

[47] F. Wöhler, *Annalen Physik Chemie*, 12, 253-256, 1828

[48] H. C. Schröder, D. Brandt, U. Schlossmacher, X. Wang, M. N. Tahir, W. Tremel, S. I. Belikov and W. E. G. Müller, *Naturwissen.*, 94, 339-359, 2007

[49] M. N. Tahir, P. Theato, W. E. G. Müller, H. C. Schröder, A. Janshoff, J. Zhang, J. Huth and W. Tremel, *Chem. Commun.*, 2848-2849, 2004

[50] M. N. Tahir, P. Theato, W. E. G. Müller, H. C. Schröder, A. Borejko, S. Faiß, A. Janshoff, J. Huth and W. Tremel, *Chem. Commun.*, 5533–5535, 2005

[51] J. L. Sumerel, W. Yang, D. Kisailus, J. C. Weaver, J. H. Choi and D. E. Morse, *Chem. Mater.*, 15, 4804-4809, 2003

[52] P. Curnow, P. H. Bessette, D. Kisailus, M. M. Murr, P. S. Daugherty and D. E. Morse, *J. Am. Chem. Soc.*, 127, 15749-15755, 2005

[53] V. Bansal, D. Rautaray, A. Ahmad and M. Sastry, *J. Mater. Chem.*, 14, 3303-3305, 2004

[54] D. Kisailus, J. H. Choi, J. C. Weaver, W. Yang and D. E. Morse, Adv. Mater., 2005, 17, 314-318

[55] M. N. Tahir, M. Eberhardt, H. A. Therese, U. Kolb, P. Theato, W. E. G. Müller, H. C. Schröder and W. Tremel, *Angew. Chem., Int. Ed.*, 45, 4803-4809, 2006

[56] M. I. Shukoor, F. Natalio, H. A. Therese, M. N. Tahir, V Ksenofontov, M. Panthöfer, M. Eberhardt, P. Theato, H. C. Schröder, W. E. G. Müller, W. Tremel, *Chem. Mat.*, 20, 3567-3573, 2008

[57] M. N. Tahir, F. Natalio, H. A. Therese, A. Yella, N. Metz, M.R. Shah, R. Berger, P. Theato, H. C. Schröder, W.E.G. Müller, W. Tremel, *Adv. Funct. Mat.*, 19, 285-291, 2009

[58] P. Curnow, D. Kisailus and D. E. Morse, *Angew. Chem., Int. Ed.*, 45, 613-616, 2006

[59] F. Natalio, E. Mugnaioli, M. Wiens, X. Wang, M.N. Tahir, W. Tremel, U. Kolb, W. E. G. Müller, *Cell Tissue Res., in press*

[60] E. Struyf, D.J. Conley, *Frontiers Ecol. Environ.-View*; doi:10.1890/070126., 2008

[61] E.M. Carlisle In: *Silicon Biochemistry*, Ciba Foundation symposium 121. Wiley, Chichester, UK, 123-139, 1986

[62] K. van Dyck, H. Robberecht, R. van Cauwenbergh, V van Vlaslaer, *Biological Trace Element. Res.*, 77, 25-32, 2000

[63] E.M. Carlisle, *Science*, 178, 619-621, 1972

[64] H.C. Schröder, A. Borejko, A. Krasko, A. Reiber, H. Schwertner, W.E.G. Müller, *J. Biomed. Mat. Res. Part B- Appl. Biomat.*, 75B, 387-392, 2005

[65] W.E.G. Müller, A. Boreiko, X.H. Wang, A. Krasko, W. Geurtsen, M.R. Custódio, T. Winkler, L. Lukić-Bilela, T. Link, H.C. Schröder, *Calcified Tiss. Internat.*, 81, 382-393, 2007

[66] D McConnell, *J. Dent. Res.*, 31, 53-63, 1952

[67] D. McConnell, *Clin. Orthopead.*, 23, 253-258, 1962

[68] W.F. Neuman, M. W. Neuman, *Chemical dynamics of Bone Mineral*, University of Chigado Press, Chicago, USA, 1958

[69] J. Y. Rho, L. Kuhn-Spearing and P. Zioupos, *Med. Eng. Phys.*, 22, 92-102, 1998

[70] J. D. Currey, *Nature*, 195, 513-514, 1962

[71] J.D. Currey, *J. Biomech.*, 37,549–556, 2004

[72] W. S. Jee, *J. Musculoskelet. Neuronal Interact.*, 1, 183-184, 2001

[73] J. M. Pachence, *J. Biomed. Mater. Res.*, 33, 35–40, 1996

[74] J. S. Nyman, A. Roy, X. M. Shen, R. L. Acuna, J. H. Tyler and X. D. Wang, *J. Biomech.*, 39, 931-938, 2006

[75] R.A. Robinson, M.L. Watson, *Anat. Rec.*, 114, 383-410, 1952

[76] W.F. de Jong, *Recl. Trav. Chym. Pays-Bas Belg.*, 45, 445-448, 1926

[77] R. Klement, G. Trömel, *Z. Physiol. Chem.*, 213, 263-292, 1932

[78] H. R. Wenk and F. Heidelbach, *Bone*, 24, 361-369, 1999

[79] G.N. Ramachandran, and G. Kartha, *Nature (London)*, 176, 593-595, 1955

[80] A.Miller, *Phil. Trans. R. Soc. London Ser. B*, 304, 455-477, 1984

[81] A.J. Hodge and J.A. Petruska In: Aspects of Protein Structure (eds G.N. Ramachradan), Academic Press, New York, 289-300, 1963

[82] S. Weiner, and W. Traub, *FEBS Lett.*, 206, 262-266, 1986

[83] J. D. Currey, *The Mechanical Adaptation of Bones*, Princeton University Press, Princeton, NJ, 1984

[84] G.W. Bernard, and D.C. Pease, *Am. J. Anat.*, 125, 271-290, 1969

[85] C.V. Gay, H. Schraer, and T.E. Hargest, *Metab. Bon. Dis. Rel. Res.*, 1, 105-108, 1978

[86] H. C. Schröder, F. Natalio, I. Shukoor, W. Tremel, U. Schloßmacher, X. Wang and W.E.G. Müller, *J. Struct. Biol.*, 159, 325-334, 2007

[87] W.J. Landis, *J. Ultrastruct. Res.*, 94, 217-238, 1986

[88] W.E. Brown, *Clin. Orthop. Rel. Res.*, 44, 205-220, 1966

[89] P.J.C. Dopping-Hepenstal, S.J. Ali, and T.C.B. Stamp In: *Matrix vesicle* (eds A. Ascenzi, E. Bonucci, and B de Bernard, Wichtig Editore, Milan, Italy, 229-234, 1981

[90] J. Sela, D. Amir, Z. Schwartz, and H. Weinberg, *Bone*, 8, 245-250, 1987

[91] R. Ampiro and E. Engström, *Acta Anat.*, 15, 1-22, 1952

[92] K. Simkiss, *Bone and Biomineralization*, Eduard Arnold Publishers Ltd, London, UK, 1975

[93] P. V. Giannoudis, H. Dinopoulos and E. Tsiridis, *Int. J. Care Injured*, 36, 20-27, 2005

[94] C.T. Laurencin, A.M.A. Ambrosio, M.D. Borden, J.A. Cooper, *Annu. Rev. Biomed. Eng.*, 1:19-46, 1990

[95] A. Bobbio, *Bull. His. Dent.*, 20, 1-6, 1972

[96] E. Lopez, B. Vidal, S. Berland, G. Camprasse, S. Camprasse, C. Silve, *Tissue Cell*, 24, 667-679, 1992

[97] O. Delattre, Y. Catonne, S. Berland, S. Borzeix and E. Lopez, *Eur. J. Orthop. Surg. Traumatol.*, 7, 143-147, 1997

[98] E. Bäuerlein and M. Epple (ed) *Handbook of Biomineralization, Vol.2: Biomimetic and Bioinspired Chemistry*, Wiley-VCH, Weinheim, Germany, 2006

[99] E. Bäuerlein and M. Epple (ed) Handbook of Biomineralization, Vol. 3: Medical and Clinical Aspects, Wiley-VCH, Weinheim, Germany 2006

[100] D. Tadic, M. Epple, *Biomaterials*, 25, 987-994, 2004

[101] J.M. Rueger, W Linhart, D. Sommerfeldt, *Orthopäde*, 27, 85-89, 1998

[102] Y. Doi, H. Iwayama, T. Shibutani, Y. Morikawa, Y. Iayama, *J. Biomed. Mat. Res.*, 47, 424-433, 1999

[103] D. Briem, W. Linhart, W. Lehman, N.M. Meenen, J.M. Rueger, *Unfallchirurg.*, 105, 128-133, 2002

Bibliography

[104] A.F. Schilling, W. Linhart, S. Filke, M. Gebauer, T. Schinke, J.M. Rueger, M. Amling, *Biomaterials*, 25, 3963-3972, 2004

[105] B.R. Constanz, I.C. Ison, M.T. Fulmer, R.D. Poser, S.T. Smith, M. VanWagoner, J. Ross, S.A. Goldstein, J.B. Jupiter, D.I. Rosenthal, *Science*, 267, 1796-1799, 1995

[106] E. Fernandez, F.J. Gil, M.P. Ginebra. F.C.M. Driessens, J.A. Planell, S.M. Best, *J. Mater. Sci. Mater. Med.*, 10, 177-183, 1999

[107] L.L. Hench, *J. Am. Ceram. Soc.*, 81, 1705-1728, 1998

[108] A.G. Mikos, A.J. Thorsen, L.A. Czerwonka, Y. Bao, R. Langer, D.N. Winslow, J.P. Vacanti, *Polymer*, 35, 1068-1077, 1994

[109] R. Langer, *Acc. Chem. Res.*, 33, 94-101, 2000

[110] R. Langer, N.A. Peppas, *Chem. Eur. J.*, 49, 2990-3006, 2003

[111] O. Böstman, H. Pihlajamäka, *Biomaterials*, 21, 2615-1621, 2000

[112] N.A. Ashammakhi, *J. Biomed. Mater. Res.*, 33, 297-303, 1996

[113] O.M. Böstman, *Clin. Orthop. Rel. Res.*, 329, 233-239, 1996

[114] E. Chiellini, R. Solaro, *Adv. Mat.*, 8, 305-331, 1996

[115] M. Vert, G. Schwarch, J. Coudane, *J. Macromol. Sci. Pure Appl. Chem.*, A32, 787-796, 1995

[116] C. Martin, H. Winet, J.Y. Bao, *Biomaterials*, 17, 2373-2380, 1996

[117] H. Winet, J.Y. Bao, *J. Biomater. Sci. Polymer Edn*, 8, 517-532, 1997

[118] C.M. Agrawal, K.A. Athanasiou, *J. Biomed. Mater. Res.*, 38, 105-114, 1997

[119] C. Schiller, M. Epple, *Biomaterials*, 24, 2037-2043, 2003

[120] L.L. Hench, H.C., Paschall, *J. Biomed. Mater. Res. Biomed. Mater. Symp.*, 4, 25-42, 1971

[121] L.L. Hench and J. Wilson In: *Silicon Biochemistry*, Ciba Foundation Symposium, Wiley, Chichester, UK, 233, 1986

[122] L.L. Hench and J. Wilson In: *Silicon Biochemistry*, Ciba Foundation Symposium, Wiley, Chichester, UK, 234, 1986

[123] L.L. Hench, A.E. Clark In: Williams DF (ed) *Biocompatibility of orthopaedic implants*. CRC Press, Boca Raton, Florida,USA, Vol: 2, Chapter 6, 129170, 1982

[124] U.M. Gross, V. Strunz In In: Lee AJC, Albrektsson T, Branemark PJ (eds) Clinical applications of biomaterials. J Wiley & Sons, New York, USA, 237-244, 1982

[125] J. Wilson, G.H. Pigott, F.J. Schoen, L.L. Hench, *J. Biomed. Mater. Res.*, 15, 805-81, 1981

[126] M. W. G. Lockyer, D. Holland, R. Dupree, *J. Non-Crys. Sol.*, 188, 207-219, 1995

[127] L. Sachs, *Angewandte Statistik*; Springer: Berlin,Germany, 242, 1984

[128] M. Nee, T. Nakamura, C. Ohtsuki, T. Kokubo and T. Yamamuro, *J. Biomed. Mat. Res.*, 27, 999-1006, 1993

[129] C. Ohtsuki, H. Kushitani, T. Kokubo, S. Kotani and T. Yamamuro, *J. Biomed. Mater. Res.*, 25, 1363-1370, 1991

[130] C. Wagner-Hülsmann, N. Bachinski, B. Diehl-Seifert, B. Blumbach, R. Steffen, Z. Pancer, W.E.G. Müller, *System. Glycobiol.*, 6,785-793, 1996

[131] A. Krasko, R. Batel, H.C. Schröder, I.M. Muler, W.E.G. Müller, *Eur. J. Biochem.*, 267, 4878-4887, 2000

[132] O. V. Kaluzhnaya, S. I. Belikov, H. C. Schröder, M. Rothenberger, S. Zapf, J. A. Kaandorp, A. Borejko, I. M. Müller and Werner E. G. Müller, *Naturwissen.*, 92, 128-133, 2005

[133] American Society for Testing and Materials (ASTM) D-2240 specification www.astm.org/

[134] T. Mosmann, *J. Immunol. Meth.*, 65, 55–63, 1983

[135] H. Nakashima, K. Omae, T. Sakai, K. Yamazaki and H.Sakurai, *Arch. Toxicol.*, 68, 277-283, 1994

[136] G. Shaw, S. Morse, M. Ararat, F.L. Graham, *FASEB J.*, 16, 8, 869-71, 2002

[137] J.Cockin, *J. Bone Joint Surg. Br.*, 53, 153-158, 1971

[138] E.M. Younger, M.W. Chapman, *J. Orthop. Trauma*, 3, 192-195, 1989

[139] Merz H, P.G. Rytik, W.E.G. Müller, W. Röder, *Unfallchirurg.*, 94: 47-49, 1991

[140] B. D. Ratner, A. S. Hoffman, J. F. Schoen, & J. E. Lemons In: *Biomaterials Science, an Introduction to Materials in Medicine*, Academic, San Diego, USA, 1-8, 1996

[141] H. Okada, H. Toguchi, *Crit. Rev. Ther. Drug Carr. Syst.*, 12, 1-99, 1995

[142] R. Langer, J. Folkman, *Nature*, 263, 797-800, 1976

[143] S. Cohen, T. Yoshioka, M. Lucarelli, L.H. Hwang, R. Langer, *Pharm. Res.*, 8, 713-720, 1991

[144] D. Hshieh, W. Rhine, R. Langer, *Pharm. Sci.*, 72, 17-22, 1983

[145] L.G. Cima, J.P. Vacanti, C. Vacanti, D. Ingber, D. Mooney, R. Langer, *J. Biomech. Eng.*, 113, 143-151, 1991

[146] G. Zhu, S. R. Mallery, and S. P. Schwendeman, *Nat. Biotechnol.*, 18, 52-57, 2000

[147] K. Fu, A.M. Klibanov and R. Langer, *Nat. Biotechnol.*, 18, 1, 24–25, 2000

[148] B.-S. Kim, C.-S. Kim, and K.-M. Lee, *Arch. Pharm. Res.*, 31, 1050-1054, 2008

[149] A.G. Andreopoulos, E. Hatzi and M. Doxastakis, *J. Mat. Sci: Mat. in Med.*, 233-239, 2001

[150] M. Isobe, T. Amagasa, S. Oida, Y. Yamazaki, K. Ishihara, N. Nakabayashi, *J. Biomed Mat. Res. Part A*, 32, 433-438, 1998

[151] F. E. Webera, G. Eyricha, K. W. Grätza, F. E. Malyb and H. F. Sailera, *Int. J. Oral Max. Surg.*, 31, 60-65, 2002

[152] O.L. Johnson, J.L. Cleland, H.J. Lee, M. Charnis, E. Duenas, W. Jaworowicz, D. Shepard, A. Shahzamani, AJ. Jones, S.D. Putney, *Nat Med.*, 2, 795-799, 1996

[153] T. Aghaloo, C.M. Cowan, Y.F. Chou, X.L. Zhang, H.F. Lee, S. Miao, *Am. J. Pathol.*, 169, 903-915, 2006

[154] D. K. Pettit, J. R. Lawter, W. J. Huang, S. C. Pankey, N. S. Nightlinger, D. H. Lynch, J. Ann, C. L. Schuh, P. J. Morrissey and W. R. Gombotz, *Pharm. Res.*, 14, 1422-1430, 1997

[155] S. Giovagnoli, P. Blasi, M. Ricci, and C. Rossi, *AAPS PharmSciTech.*, 5, 1-9, 2004

[156] E. A. Simone, T. D. Dziubla, D. E. Discher, and V. R. Muzykantov, *Biomacromolecules*, 10, 1324-1330, 2009

[157] G. Zhu and S. P. Schwendeman, *Pharm. Res.*, 17, 350-356, 2000

[158] W. Jiang and S. P. Schwendeman, *Pharma. Res.*, 18, 878-885, 2001

[159] N. Nihant, C. Schugens, C. Grandfils, R. Jérôme and P. Teyssié, *Pharma. Res.*, 11, 1479-1484, 1994

[160] T. Morita, Y. Sakamura, Y. Horikiri, T. Suzuki and H. Yoshino, *J. Contr. Rel.*, 69, 435-444, 2000

[161] P. Molyneux & H. P. Frank, *J. Am. Chem. Soc.*, 83, 3169-3174, 1961

[162] P. Molyneux & H. P. Frank, *J. Am. Chem. Soc.*, 83, 3175-3180, 1961

[162] P. Molyneux & H. P.Frank, *J. Am. Chem. Soc.*, 86, 4753-4757, 1964

[163] P. Molyneux & M. Cornarakis-Lentzos, *Col. Polym. Sci.*, 257, 855-873, 1979

[164] P. Molyneux & S. Vekayanondha, *J. Chem. Soc. Farad. Trans,* 1, 82, 291-318, 1986

[165] A.J.M. D'Souza, R.L. Schowen, R.T. Borchardt, J.S. Salsbury, E.J. Munson, E.M. Topp, *J. Pharma. Sci.*,

92, 585-593, 2003

[166] G Gaucher, M. Poreba, F. Ravenelle, J.C. Leroux, *J. Pharm. Sci.*, 96, 1763-1775, 2007

[167] G. Gaucher, K. Asahina, J. Wang, J.C. Leroux, *Biomacromolecules*, 10, 408-416, 2009

[168] J. P. Bearinger, D. G. Castner, S. L. Golledge, A. Rezania, S. Hubchak, and K. E. Healy, *Langmuir*, 13, 5175-5183, 1997

[169] N. Vlachya, D. Tourauda, J. Heilmannb and W. Kunza, *Coll. Surf. B: Biointerfaces*, 70, 278-280, 2009

[170] W. Lu, T.G. Park, *Biotechnol. Prog.*, 11, 224-227, 1995

[171] W. Lu, T.G. Park, *J. Pharm. Sci. Technol.*, 1, 13-19, 1995

[172] M. Zilberman, I Shraga, *J. Biomed. Mat. Res. A*, 79A, 370-379, 2005

[173] W. Jiangand S. P. Schwendeman, *Pharm. Res.*, 18, 878–885, 2001

[174] S. Giovagnoli, P. Blasi, M. Ricci, and C. Rossi, *AAPS PharmSciTech.*, 5, 1-4, 2004
[175] D.S.T. Hsieh, W.D. Rhine, R. Langer, *J. Pharm. Sci.*, 72, 17-22, 1983

[176] A. Lamprecht, U. Schafer, C.M. Lehr, *AAPS PharmaSciTech.*, 1, E17, 2000

[177] M. Frangione-Beebe, R. T. Rose, P. T. P. Kaumaya, S. P. Schwendeman, *J. Microencaps.: Micro and Nano Carriers*, 18, 663-677, 2001

[178] R.K. Iler, *The chemistry of silica*. Plenum Press, NewYork, USA, 1979

[179] T. Kokubo In: *Handbook of Biomineralization, Vol.3: Medical and Clinical Aspects,* E. Bäuerlein and M. Epple (ed) Wiley-VCH, Weinheim, Germany, 2006

[180] C. Denga, J. Weng, X. Lua, S.B. Zhoua, J.X. Wana, S.X. Qua, B. Fenga and X.H. Lia, *Mat. Sci. Eng.: C*, 28, 1304-1310, 2008

[181] W. Cui, X. Li, J. Chen, S. Zhou and J. Weng, *Cryst. Growth Des.*, 8, 4576-4582, 2008

Bibliography

[182] L. Clèries, J. M. Fernández-Pradas and J. L. Morenza, *Biomaterials*, 21, 1861-1865, 2000

[183] L.-C. Gerhardt, G. Jell, A. Boccaccini, *J. Mat. Sci.: Mat. in Med.*, 18, 1287-1298, 2007

[184] J. Zhang du, L.F. Zhang, Z.C. Xiong, W. Bai, C.D. Xiong, *J Mater Sci Mater Med.*, 20, 1971-1978, 2009

[185] K. Zhang, Y. Wang, M.A. Hillmyer, L.F. Francis, *Biomaterials*, 25, 2489-2500, 2004

[186] G Crotts, T.G. Park, *J. Control Releas.*, 44, 123-134, 1997

[187] T.-i. Kim, H. J. Seo, J. S. Choi, J. K. Yoon, J. Baek, K. Kim, and J.-S. Park, *Bioconjugate Chem.*, 16, 114-0-1148, 2005

[188] Y. Lim, C. Kim, K. Kim, S. W. Kim, and J. Park, *J. Am. Chem. Soc.*, 122, 6524-6525, 2002

[189] Y. Lim, Y. H. Choi, and J. Park, *J. Am. Chem. Soc.*, 121, 5633-5639, 1999

[190] K. E. Uhrich, S. M. Cannizzaro and R. S. Langer, K. M. Shakesheff, *Chem. Rev.*, 99, 3181-3198, 1999

[191] C.C. Perry, T. Keeling-Tucker, *J. Biol. Inorg. Chem.*, 5, 537-550, 2000

[192] A.L. Samuels, A.D.M. Glass, D.H. Ehret, J.G. Menzie, *Ann. Bot.*, 72, 433-440, 1993

[193] P. Ramsohoye, I. B. Fritz, *J. Cell. Physio.*,165, 145-154, 2005

[194] K. Schwarz, D.B. Milne, *Science*, 239, 333-334, 1972

[195] K. Schwarz, *Proc. Nat. Acad. Sci. USA*, 70, 1608-1612, 1973

[196] R. F. Hamilton, S.A. Thakur, J.K. Mayfair, A. Holian, *J. Biol. Chem.*, 281, 34218-34226, 2006

[197] R. Li, A. E. Clark and L. L. Hench, *J. Appl. Biomat.*, 2, 231-239, 1991

[198] I. Izquierdo-Barba, L. Ruiz -Gonzalez, J. C. Doadrio, J. M. Gonzalez-Calbet and M. Vallet-Regí, *Solid State Sci.*, 7, 983-991, 2005

Bibliography

[199] M. Colilla, M. Manzano, M Vallet-Regí, *Int. J. Nanomed.*, 3, 404-414, 2008

[200] T. Coradin, M.M. Giraud Gille, C. Helary,C. Sanchez, J. Livage, *Mat. Res. Soc. Symp. Proc.*, 725, Q5.2.1, 2002

[201] D. Eglin, K.L. Shafran, J. Livage, T. Coradin, C.C. Perry, *J. Mat. Chem.*, 16, 4220-4230, 2006

[202] I.R. Gibson, S.M. Best and W. Bonfield, *J. Biomed. Mat. Res.*, 44, 422-428, 1999

[203] C.M. Botelho, M.A. Lopes, I.R. Gibson, S.M. Best, J.D. Santos, *J. Mater. Sci. Mater. in Med.*, 13, 1123-1127, 2002

[204] A. E. Porter, T. Buckland, K. Hing, S.M. Best, W. Bonfield, *J. Biomed. Mat. Res. A*, 78, 25-33, 2006

[205] I.R. Gibson, K.A. Hing, P.A. Revell, J.D. Santos, S.M. Best and W. Bonfield, *Key Eng. Mater.*, 218-220, 203-206, 2002

[206] N. Patel, I.R. Gibson, K.A. Hing, S.M. Best, P.A. Revell, W. Bonfield, *J. Mater. Sci. Mater. in Med.*, 13, 1199-1206, 2002

[207] N. Patel, R.A. Brooks, M. Clarke, P. Lee, N. Rushton, I.R. Gibson, S.M. Best and W. Bonfield, *J. Mat. Sci. Mater. in Med.*, 16, 429-440, 2005

[208] J. C. Vogt, G. Brandes, N. Ehlert, P. Behrens, I. Nolte, P. P. Mueller, T. Lenarz, M. Stieve, *J. Biomat. App.*, 24, 175-191, 2009

[209] K.-O. Henkel, J.-H. Lenz, Th. Gerber,V. Bienengräber, *J. Implant.*, 5, 40-42, 2005

[210] Wintermantel, E., Mayer, J, Blum, K.L., Eckert, P., Luscher, P., and Mathey M., *Biomaterials*, 17, 83-91, 1996

[211] J. Elisseeff, K. Anseth, W. McIntosh, D. Sims, M. Randolph and R. Langer, *Proc. Nat. Acad. Sci. USA*, 96, 3104-3106, 1999

[212] J. S. Temenoffa and A. G. Mikos, *Biomaterials*, 21, 2405-2412, 2000

[213] R. Langer and J.P. Vacanti, *Science*, 260, 920-926, 1993

[214] J.P. Vacanti, *Arch. Surg.*, 123, 545-549, 1988

[215] B. E. Chaignaud, R.S. Langer, J.P. Vacanti, In: A. Atala, D. Mooney, J.P. Vacanti and R.S. Langer, "Synthetic Biodegradable Polymer Scaffolds", Birkhäuser Boston, USA, 1-14, 1997

[216] P. Thomsen, J. A. Hubbell, D. Williams, and R. Canceda, *Tissue engineering*, Academic Press, Elsevier, USA, 649-684, 2008

[217] D. Green, D. Walsh, S. Mann, R.O.C. Oreffo, *Bone*, 30, 810-815, 2002

[218] G. H. Bourne, *The Biochemistry and Physiology of Bone*, Academic Books Ltd. London, UK, 1956

[219] B. Robinson, J.O. Hollinger, E. Szachowicz, J. Brekke, *Otolaryngol. Head Neck Surg.*, 112, 707-713, 1995

[220] J.E. Dennis, S.E. Haynesworth, R.G. Young, A.I. Caplan, *Cell Transpl.*, 1, 23-32, 1992

[221] S.L. Ishaug, R.G. Payne, M.J. Yaszemski, T.B. Aufdemorte, A.G. Mikos, *Biotech. Bioeng.*, 50, 443-451, 1996

[222] M. Vallet-Regí, L. Ruiz-Gonzalez, I. Isquierdo-Barba and J. M. Gonzalez-Calbet, *J. Chem. Mat.*, 16, 26-31, 2006

[223] I. Ortega, M. Jobbágy, M.L. Ferrer and F. del Monte, *Chem. Mat.*, 20, 7368-7370, 2008

[224] M.N. Tahir, F. Natalio, R. Berger, M Batz, P. Theato, H.C. Schröder, W.E.G. Müller, W. Tremel, *Soft Matter*, 5, 3657-3662, 2009

[225] S. Krimm, J. Bandekar, *Adv. Protein Chem.*, 1986, 38, 181-364

[226] G. P. Roach, D. Farrar, and C. C. Perry, *J. Am. Chem. Soc.*, 128, 3939-3945, 2006

[227] D.M. Reffit, N. Osgton, R. Jugdaohsingh, H.F.J. Cheung, B.A.J. Evans, R.P.H. Thompson, J.J. Powell, and G.N. Hampson, *Bone*, 32, 127-135, 2003

[228] M. Q. Arumugam, D.C. Ireland, R.A. Brooks, N. Rushton, W. Bonfield, *Key Eng. Mat.*, 254-256, 869-872, 2004

[229] M. Wiens, X. Wang, F. Natalio, H. C. Schröder, U. Schloßmacher, W. Guersten, W.E.G. Müller, *submitted to Adv. Biomat.*

8. List of abbreviations

A

A	Ampere
Ab	Antibodies
$AuCl_4$	tetrachloroaurate anions

B

BCIP	5-Bromo-4-chloro-3-indolylphosphate
BFGF	recombinant human basic fibroblast growth factor
BMP	Bone Morphogenic Proteins
BSA	Bovine Serum Albumin

C

°C	Grade Celsius
$CaCl_2$	Calcium chloride
CaO	Calcium oxide
$Ca_{10}(PO_4)_6(OH)_2$	hydroxyapatite
cm	centimeter
CO_2	carbon dioxide
CT	Computed Tomography
CTAB	cetyltrimethylammonium bromide bromide
Cy-3	indocarbocyanine 3

D

d	days
DLS	Dynamic Light Scattering
DMEM	Dulbeccos Minimum Essential Medium
DMSO	Dimethylsulfoxide

E

	EDTA	Ethylenediaminetetraacetic acid
	EDX	Energy Dispersive X-ray spectroscopy
	ELISA	Enzyme Linked Immunosorbent Assay

F

	FCS	Foecal calf serum
	FDA	United States Food and Drug Administration Agency
	FIB	Focus ion beam
	FITC	fluorescein-isothiocyanate
	FT-IR ATR	Fourier Transform Infrared spectroscopy with attenuated total reflection

G

	g	grams

H

	HA	hydroxyapatite
	HCl	hydrochloric acid
	HEK	Human Embryonal Kidney cells
	HEPES	N-2-Hydroxyethylpiperazin-N'-2-ethansulfone acid
	H_2O	water
	hr	hour(s)
	HRP	horseradish peroxidase
	HRTEM	High-Resolution Transmission Electron Microscopy
	H_2SO_4	sulfuric acid

I

	IgG	Immunglobulin G
	IP	isoelectric point

List of abbreviations

K

KCl	potassium chloride
kDa	kilodalton
K_2HPO_4	potassium hydrogenphosphate
kV	kilovolt

L

L	liter

M

mA	milliampere
MARCO	scavenger receptors
mg	milligrams
$MgCl_2$	magnesium chloride
$Mg(OH)_2$	magnesium hydroxide
min	minute
mL	milliliter
mm	millimeter
mM	millimolar
MTT	(3-(4,5-Dimethylthiazol-2-yl)-2,5-diphenyltetrazolium bromide)

N

NaCl	sodium chloride
$NaHCO_3$	sodium hydrogencarbonate
Na_2HPO_4	sodium hydrogenphosphate
Na_2O	disodium oxide
NaOH	sodium hydroxide
Na_2SO_4	sodium sulfate
NBT	*p*-nitrotetrazolium blue
nm	nanometer

List of abbreviations

	NMR	Nuclear Magnetic Resonance
	NTA	nitrilotriacetic acid

P

	PAGE	Polyacrylamide - Gel electrophoresis
	PBS	Phosphate Buffered Saline
	PDL	periodontal fibroblasts
	PEG	poly(ethylene glycol)
	PGA	polyglycolide
	pH	potentia hydrogenii
	pKa	dissociation constant
	PLA	poly(D,L-lactide)
	PLGA	poly(lactic-co-glycolic acid)
	PLASSM	poly(D,L-lactide)-silicatein-silica-containing-microspheres
	PMMA	polymethyl methacrylate
	PMSA	Plastic-like filler matrix
	P_2O_5	pyrophosphate
	PoAb-aSILIC	polyclonal antibodies raised against recombinant silicatein
	PVA	poly(vinyl alcohol)
	PVDF	polyvinylidene Difluoride
	PVME	poly(vinyl methyl ether)
	PVP	polyvinylpyrrolidone

R

	rpm	*rounds per minute*
	RT	room temperature

S

List of abbreviations

	s	seconds
	SAM	self-assembled monolayers
	SaOS-2	cells human osteosarcoma cells
	SBF	Simulated Body Fluid
	SDS	sodium dodecyl sulfate
	SEM	Scanning Electron Microscopy
	Ser	serine
	Si-HA	silica substituted hydroxyapatite
	SiO_2	silica
	SM	sodium metasilicate
	STEM	Scannning Transmission Electron Microscopy

T

	TBS	Tris Buffered Saline
	TEM	Transmission Electron Microscope
	TEMED	N,N,N',N'-Tetramethylethylendiamine
	TEOS	tetraorthosilicate
	TiO_2	titanium oxide
	Tris	tris(hydroxymethyl)aminomethane
	Tween 20	poly(oxyethylen)20-sorbitan-monolaurate

V

	v/v	*volume per volume*

W

	w/o/w	water/oil/water
	WS_2	tungsten sulfide
	wt	weight
	w/v	weight per volume
	w/w	weight per weight

List of abbreviations

X

    XRD   X-ray diffraction

Z

    ZrO_2 zirconia

Others

%	percentage
$\gamma-Fe_2O_3$	Iron oxide
µg	micrograms
µM	micromolar
µ-CT	micro-computed tomography
2im	bifunctional 2-component implant
2D	..bidimensional
3D	tridimensional
7WD10	Chinese hamster ovary cells

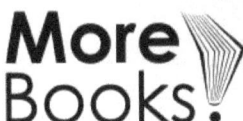
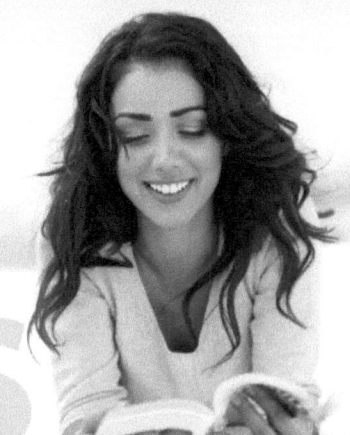

I want morebooks!

Buy your books fast and straightforward online - at one of world's fastest growing online book stores! Environmentally sound due to Print-on-Demand technologies.

Buy your books online at
www.morebooks.shop

Kaufen Sie Ihre Bücher schnell und unkompliziert online – auf einer der am schnellsten wachsenden Buchhandelsplattformen weltweit! Dank Print-On-Demand umwelt- und ressourcenschonend produziert.

Bücher schneller online kaufen
www.morebooks.shop

KS OmniScriptum Publishing
Brivibas gatve 197
LV-1039 Riga, Latvia
Telefax +371 686 204 55

info@omniscriptum.com
www.omniscriptum.com

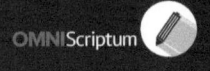

Printed by Books on Demand GmbH, Norderstedt / Germany